At

The 30 Day Guide for Shedding Weight and Living a Healthier Lifestyle

Sarah Stewart

Atkins Diet: The 30 Day Guide for Shedding Weight and Living a Healthier Lifestyle

Table of Contents

Introduction to the Atkins Diet

Do you have goals for losing weight and keeping away the pounds for years to come? At its core, weight loss involves consuming less calories than your body burns in a day. For many people, it's so much more than that. So many things get factored into the equation, such as lifestyle, genetics, medical history and attitude. Weight loss can be an emotional experience. Don't worry! There's a few things you can try to help you lose weight quickly and successfully. More importantly, there are certain diets that are designed to help you turn healthy eating into a long-term lifestyle so you can enjoy maintaining a healthy weight for years to come and avoid gaining in the future.

Healthy weight loss isn't just about eating less calories. It's about eating the right amount of vitamins, nutrients and protein that your body needs to live and thrive. Sometimes the things you eat are more important than how much or how frequently you eat. While it's important to consume food in moderation and stick to a daily calorie intake appropriate for your body, the things you put into your body are some of the primary drivers in weight loss.

This is especially true when it comes to burning fat; if you want to burn more fat in your body, what you eat matters. Burning fat by starving yourself is NOT a healthy way to lose weight. Instead, you can try a meal plan that encourages your body to target and burn fat more efficiently. One such diet is known as the Atkins diet.

The Atkins diet is a diet plan for weight loss that involves gradual changes in eating habits to promote a healthier lifestyle. The focus of the Atkins diet centers around foods that are high in protein and healthy fat, and avoiding foods that are high in carbohydrates. This is easier said than done. That's why the Atkins diet is divided up into four stages to help you transition your diet and aid your body in dealing with the changes effectively. There are four Phases, starting from eating veggie-only carbs all the way to making a balanced diet part of your lifestyle to ensure you don't gain back the weight.

I'll be showing you some tips and strategies for how to get started on your weight loss journey using the Atkins diet. I will be discussing a more flexible and healthful version of the Atkins diet so that you will be able to adapt it to your individual needs and still see results in 30 days or less. I'll also provide you with easy, simple recipes for each Phase of the Atkins diet.

Everyone has different preferences, dietary habits, special nutritional needs, and so on; that's why it's important that you find a diet plan that you can customize to your personal situation. My goal is that you can take these recipes and adapt them to your unique needs and preferences.

What is the Atkins Diet?

The Atkins diet was first introduced to the public by Dr. Robert C. Atkins, a physician and cardiologist. Dr. Atkins wrote a book in 1972 about his diet that he developed around the idea of emphasizing protein and fat while restricting carbohydrate consumption. Although his book was a best-seller, it faced a lot of controversy and his work is still criticized even after his passing in 2003. What was so controversial about the Atkins diet?

Dr. Atkin suggested that starchy carbohydrates cause people to gain weight and feel hungry. Some doctors and nutritionists argue that some forms of carbohydrates (for example, brown rice) are actually quite healthy and can help people lose weight. Additionally, consuming more protein from foods with trans fats (for example, red meat) can also cause weight gain.

You might be wondering: is the Atkins diet good for me or not? In this version of the Atkins diet that I'll be discussing, we'll still be focusing on a high protein, low carb diet but with more restrictions on trans fats and less restrictions on fiber.

The idea is to eat food that helps your body burn fat more quickly and makes you feel fuller for longer. Protein and fat will do that, but eating too much of the "wrong types" of protein and fatty foods can have counteractive results. The trick is to find a balance of protein, healthy fats and fiber to create a diet that you can stick to without consuming unhealthy carbs and excess sugar.

While the Atkins diet starts off with a high restriction on carbs, these restrictions gradually ease as the diet progresses. The initial stage is designed to jumpstart your body into losing weight through the process of ketosis, but eventually you will be able to start bringing more healthy carbs into your meals for a long-term, balanced diet to help you reach and maintain a healthy weight.

How Does the Atkins Diet Work to Help Lose Weight?

There are different variations of the Atkins diet. For example, there's the strict Atkins 20 plan and the more relaxed Atkins 40. No matter what type you might be following, the essential rules of the Atkins diet is to follow a meal plan that restricts carbs and emphasizes protein and healthy fats, with changes incorporated to the plan as weight is loss.

The secret to the Atkins diet is a natural process called ketosis. During the state of ketosis, your body is completely fueled by fat (rather than carbs). This forces your body to start burning fat, which in turn can lead to effective weight loss. Following the Atkins diet is one way you can get your body to go into ketosis and I'll be showing you some recipes that you can make during the different phases of the diet to help you see results as quickly as possible.

How do you get your body to go into ketosis and start burning unwanted fat? You have to shorten your body's supply from glucose by greatly reducing your intake of carbohydrates. Ketosis can be achieved by fasting (not eating), but that's not a healthy way of dieting! In the Atkins diet, ketosis is achieved in Phase 1 where you'll only be getting carbs from vegetables. In some cases, even protein may need to be restricted to achieve ketosis as too much protein can hinder ketosis. In addition to managing what you eat, you should also avoid snacking on junk food and only eat when you're actually hungry.

So how can you tell if it's working or not? There are a few different ways you can tell if your body is in ketosis. You can actually purchase kits from your local pharmacy or shopping center that allow you to test your own urine and get instant feedback. There are also ways to get tested with blood or breath tests, with blood-ketone meter tests being the most accurate. These tests will tell you what stage your blood ketone levels are and whether or not they're in an optimal ketosis zone. The maximum optimal level for blood ketones is about 1.5-3 mmol/l.

There are also several symptoms you can look out for if you don't want to take a test. Your body might be in ketosis if:

*You've been adamantly following the Atkins diet or a ketosis diet with high carbohydrate restrictions.

*You're feeling thirsty more often; this will be more obvious if you're not getting enough electrolytes.

*You're experiencing increased urination

*You're experiencing a reduction in hunger and an increase in energy

If you're feeling concerned about the process of ketosis, here are a few tips about the benefits and risks of going on a ketogenic diet, such as the Atkins diet:

Benefits of Ketosis

*Ketosis can help you burn fat quickly and help you lose weight

*Ketosis can possibly increase brain function

*Ketosis can possibly increase physical endurance

*Ketosis can possibly reverse type 2 diabetes

Risks of Ketosis

*Ketosis can lower insulin levels, which can be dangerous for people who suffer from insulin-related diseases

*Ketosis may cause you to experience certain side effects, such as headache or constipation. These usually only occur within the first week of reaching

ketosis, but always ask your doctor if you have concerns. Most of the side effects can be managed at home (drinking more water and eating vegetables can help with most symptoms).

If you'd like to learn more about ketosis or figure out how you can check the state of ketosis in your body, there are hundreds of free resources in the form of web pages, apps, and books that can help you get started. Tests are fairly affordable and safe, so consider buying a few if you'd like to keep a detailed record of your health during your weight loss journey. Sometimes it's interesting just to know your current ketosis zone!

Embracing Protein and Fat

Bacon, eggs, steak, cheese, butter... what's not to love? In broader renditions of the Atkins diets, these types of foods would be on the menu because they're high in proteins and fats. However, these foods also contains trans fats and cholesterol, which can lead to weight gain, inflammation, and high blood pressure. Don't worry! Delicious food full of protein and healthy fats can still be consumed on the Atkins diet.

The key is to use moderation, smart shopping and variation to help you avoid eating too much of certain foods that could hinder your weight loss. The focus will be more on lean protein (for example, chicken breast, legumes, fish, and lean beef), rather than consuming "less healthy" meats and proteins, such as fatty pork or hamburger.

You'll also be consuming more "healthy" fats and less "unhealthy" fats. Specifically, you'll be eating more foods with mono- and polyunsaturated fats as opposed to saturated and trans fats. Eating lots of fat is especially important in the process of ketosis because that's what you want your body to start burning. If you're on a low-carb diet combined with a low-fat diet, this could lead to starvation and failure to lose weight in a healthy manner.

Eating a sufficient amount of protein from foods such poultry, eggs and fish can help in the process of building and repairing cells, especially if you're looking to strengthen your muscles and organs. Consuming protein is also a great way to make you feel fuller for longer without taking in carbohydrates. That's why high-protein, low-carb diets are often successful at helping people lose weight – it's a diet that satisfies.

The bottom line – protein is critical for any weight loss diet and plays a large role in the Atkins diet (especially during the initial stages). However, a balanced diet of protein, healthy carbs (fruits, vegetables, and whole grains), and healthy fats should be the ultimate target for an overall healthy lifestyle.

Avoiding Carbohydrates (At First)

In the Atkins diet, you'll need to primarily stay away from starchy and sugary carbs. Unfortunately, these are included in many types of popular foods that people eat every day. Bread, pasta, potatoes, cookies, chips... all of these things contain carbs that can contribute to weight gain. Foods such as pizza, white bread, sugary cereals, candy and fast food can also cause you to feel hungrier and even have a negative impact on your emotions and ability to focus.

For example, a 2001 study from *Appetite* looked at the relationship between mood, cravings, and the consumption of either protein-rich food or carbohydrate-rich food. Researchers found that there was a strong correlation between people who craved carb-rich foods and the intensity of their cravings. In essence, people who craved carbs the most appeared to experience the most intense levels of cravings and mood scales.

Another example: In a 1983 study from the Journal of Psychiatric Research, Bonnie Spring and colleagues performed a study on how diet type (either high-carbohydrate or high-protein) effected the mood of human test subjects. They found that eating a high-carbohydrate, low-protein lunch caused reduced concentration, particularly in older subjects.

So, carbohydrates cravings are bad and eating carbs can impact our behavior – does that mean all carbohydrates are bad? No. Carbohydrates are sugar, starches and fibers made up of carbon, hydrogen and oxygen atoms. Our bodies use carbohydrates to obtain energy; according to the American Diabetes Association, carbohydrates are actually the body's main source of energy. So, wait a minute... we need carbs for energy? That's right, carbs play an important function in our diets and fuel for physiological processes that occur in our bodies. Remember Dr. Atkin? A lot of people criticized him because of his idea for a low-or-no carb diet. Who's right?

Not all carbs are created equal. There are two kinds of carbohydrates: simple versus complex. Simple carbs come from things candy, soda and beer; these are more easily and quickly absorbed and digested in our bodies. Complex carbs refers to the carbs found in potatoes, vegetables and whole-grains. Complex carbs take longer to digest and your body doesn't get energy from them as quickly as simple sugars; however, the energy is more sustained for a longer period of time. So which ones are "good" and which ones are "bad"?

In general, simple carbs should be avoided at all costs for weight loss. This also includes foods that are processed or contain artificial sweeteners. The "good" carbs are carbs from fruit, vegetables and whole-grains that cause your body to work more for its energy. These types of foods are lower in calories and provide additional nutrients, including fiber and antioxidants.

Still not sure how to tell which carbs you should leave alone and which ones are okay? Here are a few quick shopping tips:

Only buy carbs that are...

*Low in sodium, calories, and saturated fat

*High in nutrients and naturally occurring fiber

*Free of cholesterol, trans fats, and anything refined

*Opt for wholesome, natural ingredients. Don't get anything that comes processed from a box or states that it's a "diet" food. If it's refined or processed, you don't need it.

Never buy carbs that are...

*High in refined grains (for example, white flour), calories, sodium, sugar, saturated fats, trans fats, and cholesterol

*Low in fiber and nutrients

For the Atkins diet, most carbohydrates will be excluded from your diet plan, but not all. As you progress through the phases of the diet, you'll actually be consuming healthier, complex carbs.

The bottom line – carbohydrates are essential for fueling our bodies and helping our brains function. Choosing the healthiest carbohydrates to consume is the best way to get the vitamins, minerals and other nutrients that your body needs to survive and thrive. Don't be afraid of carbohydrates! Just learn how to tell the difference between good carbs and bad carbs – and take care to maintain your eating habits with controlled portions and wise meal choices.

A Note About Dietary Restrictions

Both vegetarians and vegans can still follow the Atkins diet by getting protein from non-meat sources, such as eggs, soy and cheese for vegetarians and legumes, nuts and seeds for vegans. However, vegans and vegetarians may need to skip the first phase of the Atkins diet because this phase greatly restricts carbs (vegans and vegetarians often need to consume larger amounts of healthy carbs compared with meat-eaters).

If you're on a sodium or gluten-restricted diet, the Atkins diet is a great option because it excludes a lot of sodium and gluten-rich carbs.

What Foods are Accepted or Restricted in the Atkins Diet?

Acceptable foods for the Atkins diet include:

Chicken and other poultry. Chicken, Cornish hen, duck, turkey, quail and other poultry is generally acceptable in the Atkins diet. Choose baking or grilling rather than frying to avoid added calories that can be counterproductive to weight loss. Season with fresh or dried herbs and spices.

Red meat. Most weight loss diets restrict red meat from beef and pork as they contain saturated fats that may cause health risks related to diabetes and heart disease (if eaten in large quantities). Stick to leaner cuts of red meat and avoid any kind of meat that's processed, sweetened or contains additives (this includes many types of bacon, ham, hotdogs and ground hamburger meat).

Fish and shellfish. Fish, especially wild-caught cold-water fish such as salmon or trout, are full of healthy protein and omega-3-fatty acids essential for weight and immune system health. Other types of fish you can try includes flounder, herring, sardines, tuna, cod and halibut. If you don't like the flavor of fish, try using less "fishy" tasting fish such as flounder or catfish. Use lots of spices and lemon juice to blend with the flavor and try different recipes to discover something you enjoy. Shellfish, such as clams, shrimp and lobster can also be part of your Atkins diet so long as you're aware of any allergies you may have to shellfish.

Eggs. While eating lots of eggs can increase your "bad" cholesterol levels, eggs are also nutrient-dense and full of protein. Eggs can be part of any healthy diet but should be limited for people with diabetes or certain disorders related to cholesterol (ask your doctor if needed). Eggs can be eaten in a variety of ways, including deviled, fried, scrambled, hard-boiled or combined with greens, herbs and cheese into an omelet. Look for pastured or Omega-3 enriched versions.

Cheese. Who doesn't love cheese? Cheese can add a depth of flavor to a variety of dishes or be eaten as a filling snack. As long as you consume cheese in moderation, there are hundreds of options to try, including parmesan, goat cheese, bleu cheeses, mozzarella, feta, cheddar and more. Note: the serving size for cheese is usually 1 ounce.

Healthy fats. Olive oil and butter are popular staples for cooking and flavoring in the Atkins diet. Use olive oil over vegetable oils and choose natural butter over margarine or "fake" butter. Mayonnaise with no added sugar can be acceptable in the Atkins diet as long as it's consumed in moderation. Serving size for these types of fats is approximately 1 tablespoon.

Vegetables. Don't be afraid to have plenty of vegetables in your diet, even in Phase 1. For best results, choose foundation vegetables such as sprouts, olives, Bok choy, lettuce, mushrooms, spinach, broccoli, avocado, onion, zucchini, cucumber, cauliflower, asparagus, bell pepper, green beans, Brussel sprouts, tomato and garlic. These types of foods will be the main carb source for Phase 1 of the diet, so use them to build around your meals containing protein and healthy fats. Remember: vegetables are important for weight loss and overall health, so be ready to use more as you progress through the diet.

Beans, legumes, and grains (in later stages). Lentils, chickpeas, quinoa, kidney beans and navy beans are a few healthy options that you can incorporate into your diet after Phase 1. Beans, legumes and grains are an excellent source of beneficial nutrients and they'll help fill you up and they make great meat substitutes. The serving size for legumes is about ¼ cup.

Dairy (in later stages). Aside from cheese, you may also consume unsweetened dairy products, such as whole milk, Greek yogurt and cottage cheese, later in the diet. For example, as opposed to non-fat or normal yogurt that has added sweeteners, use full-fat plain Greek yogurt to make dishes creamier. Full-fat dairy may contain more calories than some of the alternatives, but it won't contain any of the extra sugars or additives found in low fat versions. Full-fat products are also more satiating and can help lower the risk of diabetes. The serving size for dairy is generally ½ cup.

Nuts (in later stages). Nuts contain healthy fats and protein, so they're okay to eat with limitations in Phase 1 – in later phases, you can start eating more nuts as healthy snacks or toppings. Make sure to opt for raw, non-salted or unsweetened versions. They contain lots of calories, so keep the serving size at approximately 1 or 2 tablespoons.

Fruit (in later stages). Fruits are full of fiber and antioxidants that can benefit your whole body, from your skin to your heart. As you advance to Phase 2 and so on, you can gradually add in more fruit to your diet in the form of fresh raw fruits. The serving size of fruit is about ¼ cup.

Restricted foods for the Atkins diet include:

***Candy, soda and sugary juices**.

***White bread, white pasta, white flour, etc**.

***Potatoes, white rice and other starchy foods**

***Cakes, cookies, pastries and foods with shortening or lots of sugar and flour**

***Rice, oats and whole-wheat bread** (Phase 1 only).

If you consume any of these foods, that doesn't mean that all your progress is over. While consuming these types of food can (and will) hold you back from your goals, you should continue sticking to a low-carb diet as best as possible and don't let one stumble end your whole journey. It won't be easy, but it'll be worth it.

Is the Atkins Diet Right for Me?

Overall, anyone can try the Atkins diet and enjoy a huge variety of tasty meal options for weight loss. The Atkins diet may work best for you if you have the following qualities:

*You enjoy eating meat, seafood and eggs in your primary meals.

*You love savory foods and hearty breakfasts.

*You're able to avoid foods that are processed or contain artificial sweeteners or additives.

*You're willing to be flexible and open to new combinations.

*You feel comfortable adapting your dietary habits.

*You're in tune with your body or you're willing to keep track of changes in your weight and mood according to what you eat.

If you like the sound of eating more protein and healthy fats, eliminating junk food from your diet and losing weight as soon as possible, read on for customizable Atkins diet tips and recipes!

Chapter One: Planning and Preparation

Before going on any kind of diet, you should always talk to your doctor and make sure you're aware of any allergies you may have. Your body may have specific dietary needs that conflict with the Atkins diet, so it's important to get the "all clear" from a medical professional before moving forward. If you have diabetes or other hormonal disorders, you may experience different results during the Atkin diet process depending on how your body reacts to the different phases (especially Phase 1).

Talk to your doctor if you have diabetes or similar conditions; in some of these situations, the Atkins diet may not be appropriate. Overall, the Atkins diet is full of fresh and nutritious food that can incorporated into meals that everyone can eat to maintain a healthy lifestyle.

Now that you've been warned about any potential risk and you feel comfortable moving forward with the Atkins diet, let's begin with some tips and strategies for how to plan and prepare for a delicious and dynamic diet that's high in fats and protein and low in carbs and sugar.

Shopping Tips

When you're at the supermarket for the first time and shopping for your new diet, things can feel overwhelming. You don't want to buy the wrong things and you might be worried that you'll leave something out or end up making unhealthy choices.

Try to relax and breathe. Make sure you have something filling to eat before you go shopping to avoid having cravings that might tempt you into grabbing unnecessary snack food. Try not think about other stressful things. Instead, use this time to focus on the task at hand and avoid worrying about things that are out of your control.

Make a list. While that may seem obvious, making a detailed list before you actually go into the store can be incredibly important for staying on track with your dietary goals. Knowing exactly what you need to buy will ensure that you don't spend time scratching your head and feeling frustrated. For your first shopping trip, your list will be longer than normal because you'll probably be buying some pantry staples such as spices, herbs and oils. While you may have to pay more on your first trip, this will ultimately save you in the long run because you'll be able to make a wider range of delicious, healthy recipes and avoid turning to fast food when you don't know what to make.

Shop on the edges of the store. This includes the produce section, the meat and seafood section and areas that have fresh and unprocessed foods (note: processed foods can still be found here, so use caution and read labels – look for foods with as little ingredients as possible). The idea is to stay away from the center isles filled with products chocked full of carbs, sodium, and sugar. Exceptions include the spice and cooking isle for seasoning and olive oil.

Consider your preferences. You can buy all the kale and fish in the store but it won't do you any good if you're not going to eat it. Planning on eating healthier is all well and good, but the true key to actually losing weight is sticking to a diet that you don't hate. Chances are, you have more options than you think. Consider the wide range of ways you can prepare, season, marinate and cook lean meats, seafood, tofu, legumes, and so on. It might take some trial and error, but eventually you should be able to find something that works to your tastes without straying away from the diet.

What You'll Need to Begin

For the Atkins diet, there are several tools you'll need (or at least tools that would be very helpful) for your ultimate weight loss success. Let's get started!

A digital scale. If you're trying to lose weight, you're going to need a reliable digital scale with fresh batteries. An important component of the Atkins diet is monitoring your weight loss; not just how much you're losing, but how fast and how frequently. A scale is a tool to help you track and monitor your progress, not weigh you down or dissuade you.

Stepping on the scale, especially every day, can get emotional for some people. You might start to feel upset if you don't see immediate changes or you notice that you've started to gain even after trying hard to stick to the diet. There are many factors that affect your weight and weight can fluctuate through the day, week, month and year. The important first step is to get to know your body better. Calculate your BMI (Body Mass Index) and use it to help you plan your healthy goal weight. The scale will help you stay on track and, in the case of the Atkins diet, guide your dietary decisions. For example, you'll need to track your level of weight loss in Phase 3 to learn how many carbs you can incorporate into your diet without regaining the weight you've lost. The scale is your friend!

If you do have problems with using a scale, go ahead and disregard it for Phase 1 of the Atkins diet. The induction phase is when you may see a lot of fluctuations in your weight, so it may be best to check in after two weeks of starting Phase 1 after your body has had some time to adjust to the changes.

Food scales or an understanding of food portion sizes. Understanding grams, ounces and tablespoons in terms of food is important in successful dieting. You may be eating all of the right foods, but if you're eating too much or too little of something, you may not see the results you're hoping for. Additionally, you'll benefit from investing in a meat thermometer so you can save time and stress in situations where you're cooking meat and confused about whether or not it's fully cooked.

A solid schedule. If you have a chaotic schedule, now would be a great time to start adopting a more solid routine. Breakfast will likely be the most important meal of the day for people on the Atkins diet. This is where you're going to get your fill of protein and energy to help drive you through the first part of the day until your lunch or snack break. Start out by having a set time after you get up to eat breakfast, and stick to it. Additionally, going to bed at the same time and getting a solid 6 to 8 hours of sleep will also be highly beneficial for your weight loss regime.

Self-motivation. If you've tried other diets and you've had little success at losing weight, you're probably already feeling frustrated and worried that things won't work out. Try to think positive and focus on your goals. Not only look forward to the future but also take some time to enjoy the moment – relax in the sun, read a good book, play a game with your family. Do healthy things that you enjoy and try to rewire your perspective on dieting.

Self-control. If you're used to eating lots of fast food, bread, pasta, chips, and sugary or salty snacks, you'll need to be ready to cut back on those types of foods for this diet. If you're prone to cravings for carbs, the best way to fight them is to follow the Atkins diet as closely as possible – and stick with it!

This is because you'll be teaching your body how to run without these types of foods and feel full without the need for starchy or sugary meals. The first couple of days might be difficult, but as long as you stay strong and consistent, you should start feeling changes in your body and reductions in cravings by the end of the first two weeks.

By this time, your body will be working on burning fat and your appetite will likely be more suppressed with your protein and fat-rich meals. If you're really prone to snacking, make sure to have healthy snacks ready to grab as soon as you need them so you won't be tempted to stop at a convenience store or vending machine. Drinking lots of water throughout the day is another great way to hammer down on the cravings and keep you filled up between meals.

Chapter Two: Phase 1 Tips and Recipes

Starting Your Journey to a Happier, Healthier You

Phase 1 of the Atkins diet involves transforming your body into a fat burning machine. You'll be building your meals around protein (meat, seafood, tofu, eggs) and fats (butter, olive oil, cheese, avocados). You can pair leafy greens with your meals and eat fruit very minimally, but you should absolutely avoid bread, pasta, potatoes and most baked goods. Don't worry – Phase 1 can last as little as two weeks! If you follow the plan closely and cut out all unhealthy carbs (while dually avoiding "bad" fats and too much protein), you'll likely see changes in your weight fairly quickly.

Take your time with Phase 1; don't try and rush your body through the process of entering ketosis. You will likely experience heavy cravings during this time, so be patient and stick to the low-carb diet as closely as possible. As this is one of the most challenging parts of the diet, here are some ground rules to help you get started:

*Only eat 20 grams or less of carbs per day. The majority of that (about 15 grams) should be from vegetables. That's probably a huge drop for the average person. According to Mayo Clinic, Americans can generally eat 225 to 325 grams of carbs per day for a daily diet of 2000 calories.

This rule is flexible depending on your individual dietary needs. Your age, activity levels, body composition, metabolic health and gender all play a role in how many carbs you should eat per day, regardless of what diet you may be on. For the Atkins diet, consuming more than 20 grams of carbs may be appropriate if you're an extremely active person. If you don't want to exclude vegetables and fruit from your diet, you can actually skip this phase or modify it to be lenient for your needs. As long as you're avoiding carbs that are full of sugar, processed grains, vegetable oil and trans fats, you should see results.

*Don't be afraid to eat vegetables during this phase, but try to stick to leafy green vegetables, such as spinach and kale, as your primary source of carbs. In many versions of the Atkins diet, fruit is completely restricted during this phase, so exclude fruits if you feel that is what's best for your individual body and needs.

*Eat when you need to and never skip meals. You can either eat three regular sized meals or four or five smaller sized meals each day. Drink lots of water throughout the day to help curve your hunger. Snack ideas include cucumber slices with cream cheese spread, cherry tomatoes, lunch meat rolled with hard cheese or celery sticks with an unsweetened dip. Make sure all of your main meals include some type of protein, whether that be chicken, seafood, eggs or tofu.

*Adjust as needed and stay strong. You're well on your way to kick-starting your weight loss goals!

Breakfast

Cheesy Omelet with Avocado

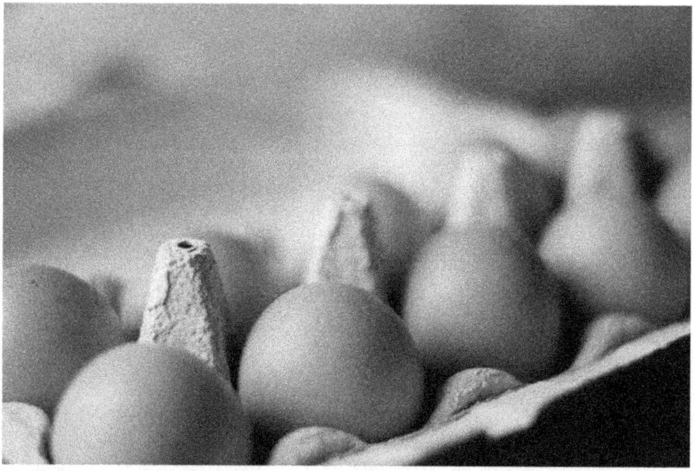

Eggs are one of the most versatile foods on the planet, and there's nothing like making a savory and convenient omelet in the morning to save time and fill you up. You can do just about anything with an egg omelet; for the Atkins diet, you can add in cheese with something green, such as asparagus, avocado or Swiss chard.

Ingredients

2 eggs (large)

1 tablespoon coconut oil or butter

2 tablespoons of water

½ avocado

1 serving pepper jack or cheddar cheese

1 tablespoon salsa (for topping)

Steps

Step One: Beating the Eggs

Start off by cracking two eggs into a bowl and adding 2 tablespoons of water. Add salt and pepper to taste and whisk the eggs with a fork or hand whisk until the whites and yolks are thoroughly blended together.

Step Two: Making the Omelet

Get out a nonstick skillet and pour in a tablespoon of butter or coconut oil, depending on your preference. Heat the skillet on medium-high and note that the oil or butter will get hot very quickly. Once the butter has melted, pour in the egg mixture. You'll see that the mixture should start to set immediately. Grab your spatula and gently pull all of the sides of the mixture toward the center. When the edges are set but the inside is still soft, you're ready to add your filling ingredients. For this recipe, just add cheese.

Step Three: Serving

While the omelet is still in the skillet, fold one side inwards and then tilt the skillet to fold the rest of the omelet over. When you put it on your plate, you want it to be have the folded side facing down. Add more pepper and sprinkle a little bit of shredded cheese on the top. Serve with a dollop of salsa and a little bit of chopped avocado.

Tips

For the filling, you can use a cup of Swiss chard or half a cup of asparagus chopped in half. Alternatively, you can use a combination of feta and spinach or add in a serving of chopped Canadian bacon for added flavor.

Scrambled Eggs with Salmon

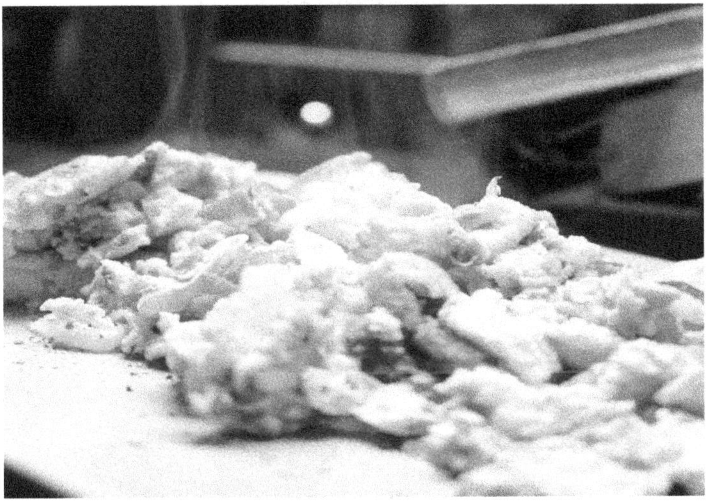

Scrambled eggs is a no-brainer if you're looking for something super simple yet filling and easy to eat. To take things up a notch, try this recipe that includes delicious salmon chunks mixed in with scrambled eggs for a unique, filling meal for breakfast or brunch.

Ingredients

4 eggs

1 tablespoon milk or heavy cream

Salt and pepper to taste

1 tablespoon butter

¼ pound smoked salmon, sliced OR ½ pound sautéed salmon fillet cut into cubes

Dill or chive to taste (optional)

Steps

Step One: Starting the Eggs

In a small bowl, whisk together the eggs, milk or heavy cream, salt and pepper. Meanwhile, melt the butter in a nonstick skillet on medium high heat. When the butter is melted, add in the egg mixture and use a wooden spoon or spatula to push around the eggs.

Step Two: Adding the Salmon

While the cooking eggs still have a wet texture, add in the salmon. You can use canned, smoked or cooked salmon chunks according to your preference. Stir the salmon into the eggs and continue scrambling them until they're cooked to your liking.

Step Three: Serving

Pour onto a plate and top with a teaspoon or so of chopped chives or dill. You can also put a little more smoked salmon on top for added garnish. In later phases of the Atkins diet, you can try this dish with whole wheat toast (for Phase 1, exclude the toast). For added richness, this dish also goes well with a little bit of mashed avocado (just make sure you're aware of your calorie intake needs).

Tips

Salmon is a great protein star in other breakfast recipes. Try smoked salmon with cream cheese and sliced cucumber for a crunchy-creamy mashup. You can also use canned salmon instead of fresh if you're on a budget.

Steak and Eggs

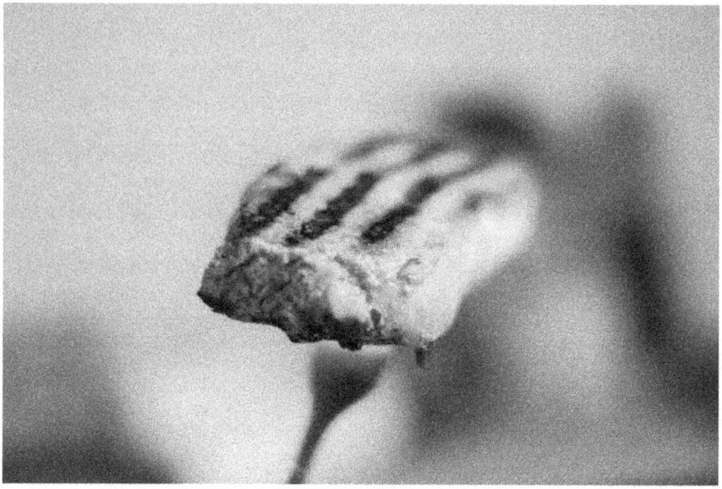

That's right, this is the kind of diet that allows you to have steak and eggs for breakfast! If you really want something to make you feel fuller for longer and help fight mid-morning cravings, try this protein-rich dish.

Ingredients

8 ounces of flank steak (avoid cuts of steaks with excess amounts of fat or trim if needed)

1 tablespoon olive oil or butter

2-4 eggs

1 ounce of shredded cheese (pepper-jack works well)

1 tablespoon salsa (for topping)

Steps

Step One: Cooking the steak

In a large nonstick skillet, heat butter until foaming and melted on high heat. Season the steak with salt and pepper to your liking and place in the skillet. Instead of putting butter in the pan, you can also coat the steak with cooking spray (just make sure to choose butter-based cooking sprays without additives). Reduce the heat and cook the steak for about 15 minutes, turning as needed to brown both sides. Alternatively, you can sear the steak on high heat and then transfer it to an oven preheated to 350 degrees Fahrenheit. Cook it in the oven for about 5 minutes until desired doneness (use a meat thermometer). Once the steak is cooked, put it onto a cutting board to rest and wipe out the excess juices from the skillet.

Step Two: Cooking the Eggs

Using the same skillet, cook the eggs in any way you'd like. To cook them sunny side up, simply crack the eggs into a skillet heated to high heat for about 3 minutes. Scrambled also pairs well with the steak.

Step Three: Serving

Slice the steak thinly against the grain and transfer a 3-4 ounce portion size to a plate. Refrigerate the rest for another meal. Top with the eggs, shredded cheese and salsa.

Tips

While this meal is rich in protein and contains healthy fats, you should try and limit your intake of red meat as much as possible. During later phases of the Atkins diet, this dish pairs well with whole-grain tortillas.

Lunch and Snacks

Baked Chicken with Broccoli

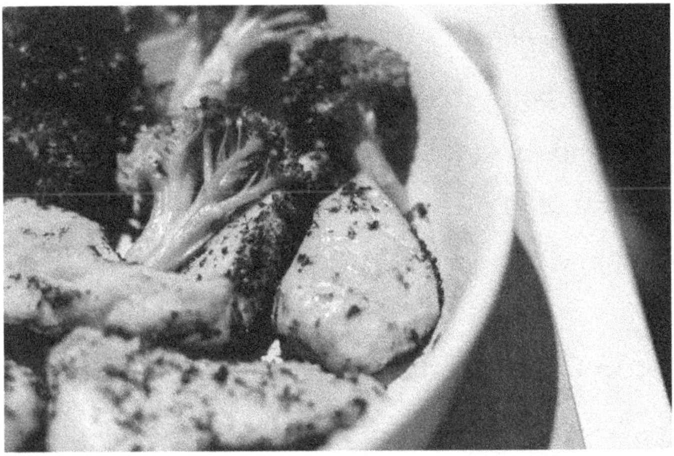

While baked chicken breasts and broccoli may not sound like the most exciting meal in the world, its versatility and health benefits for weight loss makes it a great addition to the Atkins diet. You don't have to eat it plain; you can add in other ingredients to flavor it up the way you want! However, if you're on a budget and a time crunch, there's nothing easier than baking chicken and veggies to have ready whenever hunger strikes.

Ingredients

For the chicken:

2 chicken breasts, skinless and boneless

2 tablespoons olive oil

Salt and pepper to taste

For the broccoli:

1 head broccoli, cut into florets

2 tablespoons olive oil

1 teaspoon lemon juice

1 clove of garlic

Salt and pepper to taste

Steps

Step One: Preparing the Ingredients

Preheat the oven to 400 degrees Fahrenheit. You can choose to cook the chicken and broccoli on one pan, or cook the chicken separately on a broiler pan and the broccoli on a baking sheet. Slice the chicken breasts in half down the sides so you get four thinner slices of chicken breast halves. Season with salt and pepper and rub them with olive oil on both sides. Making sure to wash your hands after touching the chicken, take the broccoli florets and toss them in a bowl with olive oil, salt, pepper, lemon juice and garlic.

Step Two: Baking

Spread the chicken and broccoli on a baking sheet in an even layer. The chicken should take about 10 minutes to bake on the first side; after that, flip the chicken and cook for another 15 minutes. Use a meat thermometer to tell when the chicken is done (it should read 165 degrees Fahrenheit). The broccoli will take about 15 to 20 minutes, depending on how tender you like them.

Step Three: Serving and Storage

Once you've removed the chicken and broccoli from the oven, allow to cool and distribute into individual portions (about 4 ounces of chicken with a half a cup of broccoli). Squirt a little bit of lemon juice on top for extra flavor. In later phases of the Atkins diet, pair the chicken with brown rice or quinoa.

Tips

Choose one day of the week to bake a few chicken breasts and distribute the chicken into individual portion sizes to eat throughout the week. Cooked chicken lasts in the fridge for 3 to 4 days, so freeze portions as needed. Instead of broccoli, try the chicken with Brussel sprouts or asparagus.

Salad with Hard Boiled Egg

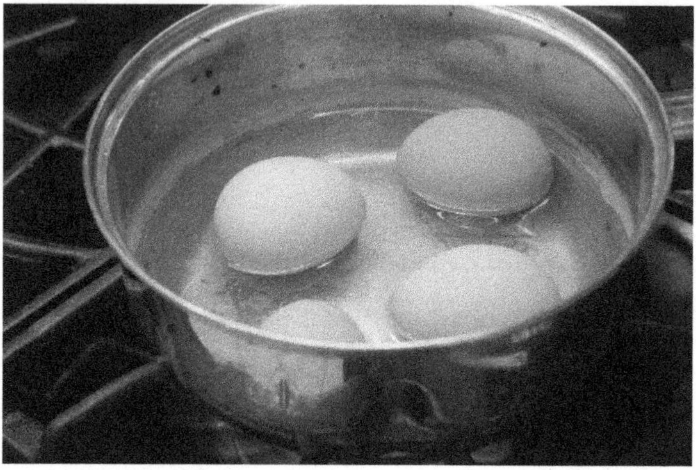

While vegetables do contain carbs, they're also rich in nutrients and fiber, and they're a key part of any diet, even the Atkins diet. Have a couple cups of this salad and top it with a protein or a healthy fat for a filling, nutritious lunch.

Ingredients

2 eggs

2 cups lettuce

½ cucumber, sliced

1 handful radishes, sliced

1 stalk celery, cut into pieces

1 tablespoon full-fat dressing (without sugar)

1 teaspoon lemon juice

Steps

Step One: Boiling the Eggs

The easiest way to boil eggs is to put them in a pot and cover them with cold water, making sure to put in the eggs first so they don't crack. Bring the pot to a rolling boil on high heat. As soon as you have a rolling boil, take the pot off the burner and cover with a lid. This is when the eggs are actually cooked. The eggs should sit in the hot water, covered, for about 15 to 17 minutes, with larger eggs needing more time. Once cooked, drain the water from the eggs and let them sit in a bowl of ice water to cool them down – do this for an hour or so if you want to have an easier time peeling them.

Step Two: Making the Salad

Using a cutting board and a sharp knife, carefully chop all of the vegetables into bite sized pieces according to your preference. Mix the vegetables together and toss in your choice of dressing and the lemon juice. Make sure the dressing you use is sugar free.

Step Three: Serving

Serve two cups of the salad into a bowl and top with one or two boiled eggs or your choice of protein. If you're not feeling like eggs, try the salad with avocado or boiled chicken as a topping instead.

Tips

Hardboiled eggs can be combined with veggies or used as a salad topping for dinner. You can also eat them as a snack by themselves.

Chicken Broth

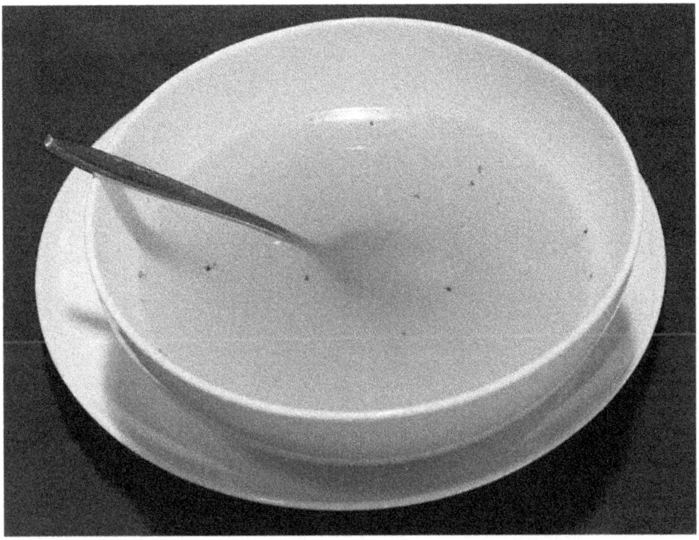

Broth can sometimes be very simple or very complex to make, depending on if you'd like to go homemade or not. Chicken or beef broth is a great low-calorie meal that you can eat when you're feeling like you're craving something salty and savory. This recipe is as simple as throwing everything in one pot and cooking with little supervision needed.

Ingredients

1 whole chicken, fat and giblets removed

2 celery stocks

6-8 baby carrots or 3-4 medium carrots

1 onion

2-3 garlic cloves

1 teaspoon peppercorns

12-16 cups of water (as needed)

Salt and pepper to taste

Steps

Step One: Preparing the Ingredients

Cut the celery stocks in half. Peel and quarter the onion. If you're using medium carrots, cut them in quarters. Gather everything together and get out a large cooking pot. Place all the ingredients, chicken first, in the pot and fill with water until just covering the chicken with an inch or two above.

Step Two: Cooking

Heat the pot on medium high heat and bring to a boil. At this point, you'll want to reduce it to a simmer. You may need to skim the fat from the surface using a spoon Allow the pot to simmer for one to 1 1/2 hours. Make sure the chicken is cooked through.

Step Three: Making the Broth

Remove the chicken and cut away the meat. Allow the chicken to cool and store the meat for salads, snacks and other meals. Continuing simmering the broth and add in the bones and carcass from the chicken. Simmer for an hour and remove from heat, allow to cool (it should get to room temperature before being stored). Discard the bones and strain the broth. Let cool and store in the fridge for 6-7 days of freeze for up to 3 months.

Tips

For added flavor, include a couple of bay leaves and some fresh thyme in the cooking process. One cup of chicken broth is a delicious and soothing low-calorie lunch or snack, especially on cold days.

Chicken and Vegetable Stir-fry

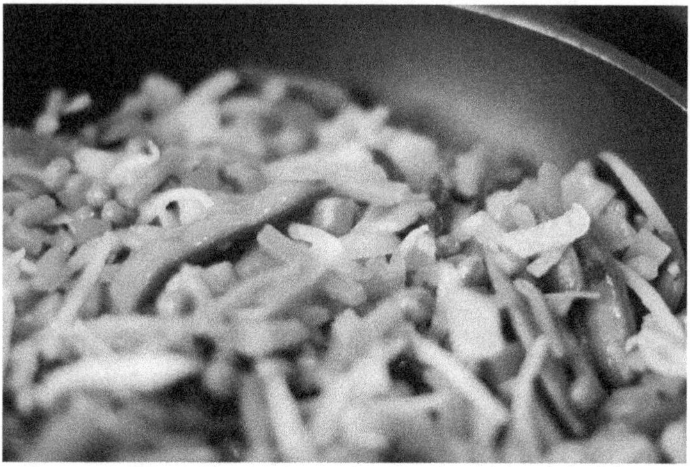

On a busy weeknight, the last thing you probably want to do is spend a long time in the kitchen conjuring up a filling, healthy meal. With this stir-fry recipe, you can cook everything in one pan and make as large or small a portion as you want. Best of all, it is low-carb if eaten without rice and also makes great leftovers.

Ingredients

2 boneless skinless chicken breasts

2 tablespoons peanut oil or olive oil

2 cups mixed frozen vegetables

½ small onion, minced

1-2 garlic cloves, minced

1 tablespoon of ginger, freshly minced

1 tablespoon low sodium soy sauce

Salt and pepper to taste

Steps

Step One: Cooking the Chicken

Cut the chicken breast into bite sized pieces and season with salt and pepper. Heat ½ tablespoon of oil in over medium high heat and cook the chicken, stir frying for about 5 or 6 minutes until the chicken is cooked through. Once cooked, set the chicken aside and save the pan for the vegetables.

Step Two: Cooking the Vegetables

Heat ½ tablespoon of oil over medium-high heat and add in the onions and garlic. Once translucent and fragrant, add in the frozen vegetables and cook for 3 or 4 minutes until tender yet crispy on the edges.

Step Three: Serving

Add back in the chicken and soy sauce to the vegetables and toss together. For added flavor, allow the stir fry to simmer, but make sure that the sauce is well distributed. Divide the stir fry into four separate servings and enjoy or store in the fridge for 3 to 4 days.

Tips

This stir-fry tastes great by itself, but in later phases of the Atkins diet, this recipe goes well with cooked brown rice or quinoa. You can also add in more flavorings, such as natural honey, fish sauce, hot sauce and even peanut butter (just make sure to use in moderation).

Coconut Garlic Spice Prawns

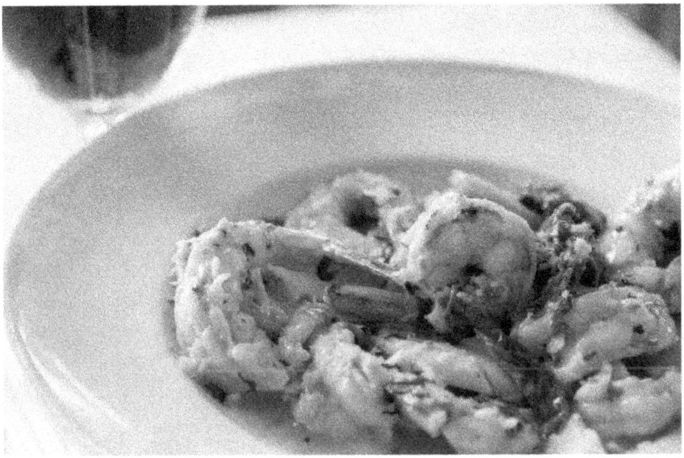

Shrimp and prawns can be used in a wide range of dishes, from creamy shrimp in soup to spicy pepper shrimp. Shrimp and other shellfish are very low-calorie, low-carb foods that can be eaten in Phase 1 of the Atkins diet. Try this sweet, low-carb recipe for coconut prawns.

Ingredients

16 ounces raw prawns or shrimp (without shell, deveined)

4-6 garlic cloves, minced

½ teaspoon curry powder

½ teaspoon chili powder

½ teaspoon red pepper flakes

1 tablespoon coconut oil

¼ coconut milk

1 tablespoon fresh parsley or chopped green onions

1 teaspoon lemon juice

Steps

Step One: Cooking the Prawns

Heat a large nonstick skillet on medium heat with 1 tablespoon coconut oil. Add in the minced garlic and cook until fragrant, stirring frequently. Clean the prawns and pat dry with a paper towel, then add the prawns into the skillet. Season the prawns with chili powder, chili flakes and curry powder. Cook the prawns until they turn pink.

Step Two: Adding the Coconut Milk

Once the prawns turn pink, pour in the coconut milk. Continue cooking until the milk begins to bubble. Add salt and pepper as needed.

Step Three: Serving

Remove the prawns from heat and serve warm with a little bit of fresh parsley or green onions and a squirt of fresh lime juice. You can also add in cooked vegetables (just add them to the skillet with the shrimp until heated through).

Tips

If you want coconut shrimp with a crunch, pan fry shrimp that's been dipped in egg and dried coconut on medium-high heat in an oiled skillet.

Grilled Fish with Green Beans

Ingredients

2 tablespoons olive oil

2 fillets of halibut, cod or other white fish of your choice

1-2 tablespoons lemon juice

1 tablespoon chopped fresh parsley

1 teaspoon dried thyme leaves, chopped

1 garlic clove, minced

1 bag frozen or fresh green string beans

2 tablespoons butter

Salt and pepper to taste

Steps

Step One: Marinating and Grilling the Fish

Mix together 1 tablespoon of olive oil, the lemon juice, thyme and garlic together in a bag. Season the fish with salt and pepper and put into the bag with the marinade. Set the bag into the fridge and allow to marinate an hour. When you're ready to cook it, heat your grill to high and put a little bit of oil on the grate (if you're dealing with extra flaky fish, you may need to use a grill basket). Cook the fish for about 4 minutes on both sides until cooked through. The fish should flake easily with a fork.

Step Two: Cooking the Green Beans

In the meantime, put one tablespoon of olive oil in a skillet heated to medium-high. Add in the green beans. Using a fresh lemon, add at least 1 teaspoon of lemon zest. Season as needed and cook for about five minutes. You want the green beans to be tender yet crisp.

Step Three: Serving

Divide the fish fillet into serving sizes (about 6 ounces cooked), and serve with green beans. Add butter on top of the fish and green beans for added richness and flavor. Garnish with fresh parsley.

Tips

White fish tastes great with many other types of sautéed or roasted vegetables if you don't like green beans. If you don't have an outdoor grill, you can bake the fish for 15 to 20 minutes at 375 degrees Fahrenheit.

Stuffed Parmesan Mushrooms (Vegetarian)

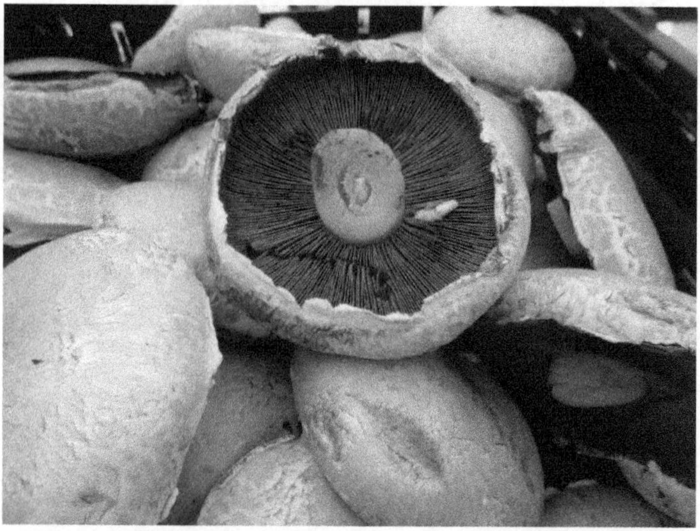

Feeling like a meatless meal for dinner? Whether you're vegetarian or just taking a break from meat, mushrooms are a delicious, meaty substitute that you can serve while also avoiding packing on the calories.

Ingredients

1 tablespoon coconut oil or olive oil

4 large portabella mushrooms

2-3 sundried tomatoes, diced

2 cups baby spinach, cut into bite sized pieces

2-3 garlic cloves, minced

½ sweet onion, diced into pieces

1/3 cup grated Parmesan

¼ feta cheese or mozzarella

Salt and pepper to taste

Steps

Step One: Preparing the Mushrooms

Clean the mushrooms thoroughly using a damp paper towel to wipe the entire mushroom. Trim the stalks (you can eat the stem if you choose). Use a spoon to remove the gills on the underside of the mushroom (you can also eat these if you want).

Step Two: Making the Filling

In a pan over medium high heat, add in the oil and sauté the onions. After about 3 minutes, add in the tomatoes and cook for another minute or two. As the onions the onions become translucent, add in the garlic, cook until fragrant, and then add in the baby spinach. Once all the ingredients are tender and the spinach is melted, remove from heat. Add seasonings and Parmesan into the mixture and generously and evenly stuff the mushrooms.

Step Three: Baking

While you're working on the ingredients, preheat your oven to 375 degrees Fahrenheit. Once you've stuffed your mushrooms, set the mushrooms onto a baking sheet and bake for about 30 minutes. Open up the oven and put the feta or mozzarella cheese on top and continue cooking for another 10 minutes or until the cheese is melted and slightly golden.

Tips

There are lots of options for stuffing mushrooms – you can even dice up small mushrooms and use those in the stuffing. You can also use dried whole wheat breadcrumbs, but avoid this during the first phase of the Atkins diet. For extra flavor, add in a tablespoon of balsamic vinegar or Worcestershire sauce into the mixture before baking.

Dessert

Sugar Free Jell-O Dessert

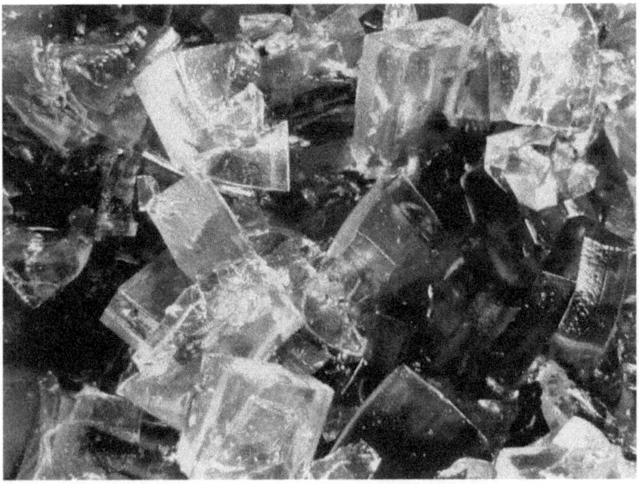

Zero-to-low carb desserts are few and far between, so you may have to suppress your sweet tooth for the first week or two of Phase 1 of the Atkins diet. Sugar free Jell-O is a common dessert eaten in the early phases of a low carb diet. To take things up a notch, make Jell-O into interesting molds and top with whipped cream. If gelatin isn't your style, you can dip fresh strawberries in melted dark chocolate, refrigerate and enjoy in moderation.

Chapter Three: Phase 2 Tips and Recipes

Start Shedding Weight Fast or at Your Own Pace

After you've made a strong effort to reduce the majority of carbs from your diet in stage one, you can start slowly bringing them back in during Phase 2. This should mainly be in the form of hearty, non-starchy vegetables and fresh fruits. If you don't mind losing weight more slowly, you're vegetarian or you just don't want to be as limited on your food choices, you can actually start the Atkins diet at Phase 2. While you may not see as rapid results as you would with Phase 1, you'll still be making great steps toward a healthier lifestyle by choosing to have a diet that's low in carbohydrates.

This is a time where you can proceed forward at your own pace. If you're not seeing the results you'd like, you may not have entered ketosis and it may be beneficial to continue excluding carbs from your diet as needed. Gradually increase your carb intake (in the form of fruits and vegetables) and see what your body's limit is in terms of what you can lose and when you stop losing. Keep in mind that the more physically active you are, the more room you have to introduce a variety of healthy carbs into your diet.

Breakfast

Turkey Sausage with Egg and Veggies

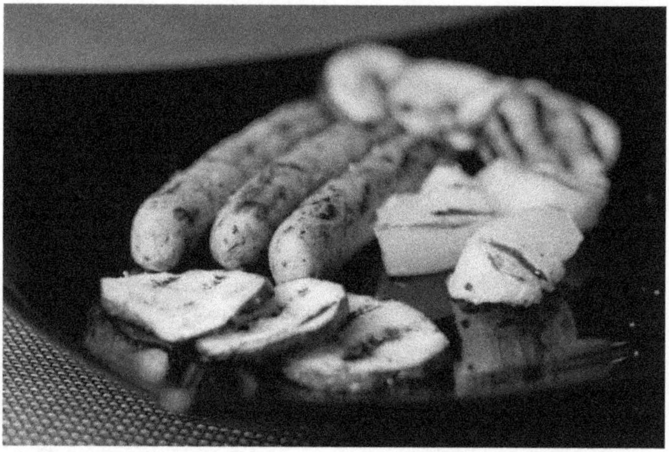

Turkey sausage can be a healthy alternative to typical pork breakfast sausage as long as you find or make some that has no sugar added with minimal sodium content. It also goes great with both sweet and savory ingredients, from peppers to apples.

Ingredients

2 turkey sausage links

1 egg

1 green bell pepper or zucchini, chopped

¼ medium onion, diced

1 orange

Pepper to taste

Steps

Step One: Cooking the Sausage

Fry the sausages in a skillet on medium heat for about one minute. Add in the onions and bell pepper and cook until the vegetables are soft and the sausage is browned. Make sure to drain excess fat as needed.

Step Two: Cooking the Egg

Cook the egg any way you'd like. You could scramble it and mix it in with chopped sausage or top the sausage with a whole, over-easy egg. Use the same skillet that you cooked the sausage in to save time.

Step Three: Serving

Serve the sausage on a plate with the vegetables and egg. You can also melt a little bit of shredded cheese on top or top with salsa depending on your preference. You can also eat this with a side of fresh fruit, such as an orange or some grapefruit.

Tips

This is a very fast breakfast meal that can also be wrapped in a whole wheat tortilla and taken on the go.

Protein Pancakes

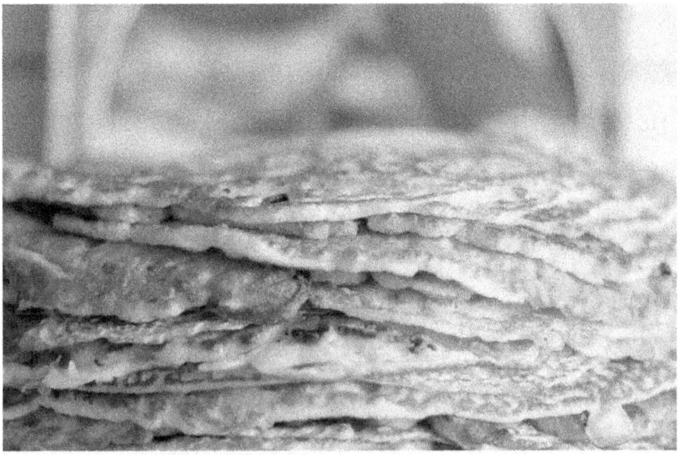

Whether you're still a kid or not, pancakes are always a hit. Luckily, there are several ingredients you can use to substitute the high carb components of pancakes, without sacrificing all of the delicious flavor.

Ingredients

3 large eggs

1 cup almond flour or coconut flour

1/3 cup protein powder or 1-2 scoops

1 teaspoon baking powder

½ tablespoon sugar substitute (optional)

1 tablespoon butter

1/3 cup cottage cheese

Steps

Step One: Make the Batter

Mix the dry ingredients (almond or coconut flour, protein powder, baking powder and sugar substitute) in a large mixing bowl. Now mix in the wet ingredients: the eggs and the cottage cheese.

Step Two: Cooking the Pancakes

Heat a nonstick skillet on medium heat. You can also use a griddle. Melt the butter in the skillet. Using a ¼ cup, scoop the pancake mixture and drop into the skillet. Cook until the pancake begins to bubble in the middle. Flip the pancakes with a spatula and cook until firm, about two minutes.

Step Three: Serving

After cooking the rest of the batter and finishing the pancakes, serve on a plate and top with a little bit of butter. Allow the leftovers to cool to room temperature and store in the fridge for up to three days or freeze for up to two months.

Tips

If you prefer, substitute the cottage cheese with cream cheese or Greek yogurt. You can also make a greater-carb but also nutritious version of these pancakes by using oats instead of flour and banana as a sweetener.

Tart Green Protein Smoothie

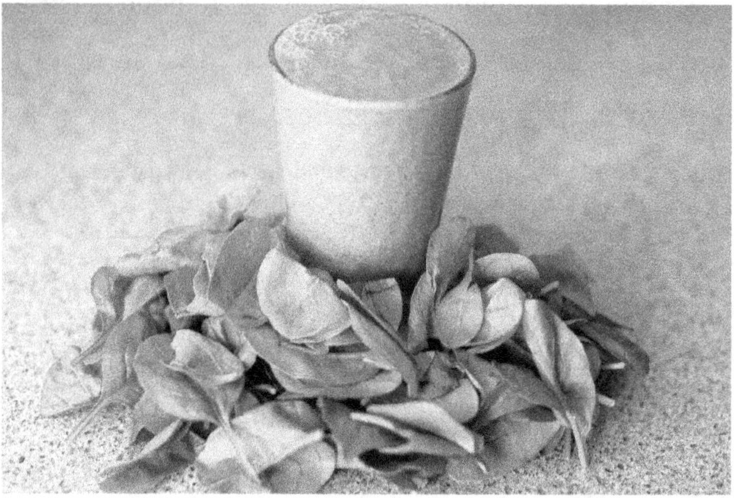

Green smoothies and juices are all the rage for low calorie, protein-packed breakfasts that you can make and drink even on your busiest days. If you're willing to give it a try, you may be pleasantly surprised by how refreshing these drinks can be.

Ingredients

½ cup ice

1-2 scoops protein powder

1 handful baby spinach

1 tablespoon lemon juice

1 cup unsweetened almond milk or whole milk

1 teaspoon vanilla extract

Steps

Step One: Preparing the Ingredients

Measure out the ingredients or set everything out so you can add as you go. Provided you have a high powered blender, you can use whole ice cubes and you don't need to worry about chopping the spinach.

Step Two: Blending

Blend all the ingredients in a high powered blender. Make sure to put in all the liquid ingredients first, followed by the firmer ingredients with the ice on top.

Step Three: Serving

Serve cold, immediately. If it's too runny for your liking, you can add in a tablespoon of chia seeds or Greek yogurt.

Tips

Try green smoothies with a variety of low calorie ingredients and get creative as you'd like. You can even use things like avocado, lime juice and heavy cream if you want something more smooth and savory.

Lunch and Snacks

Chef's Salad with Bacon

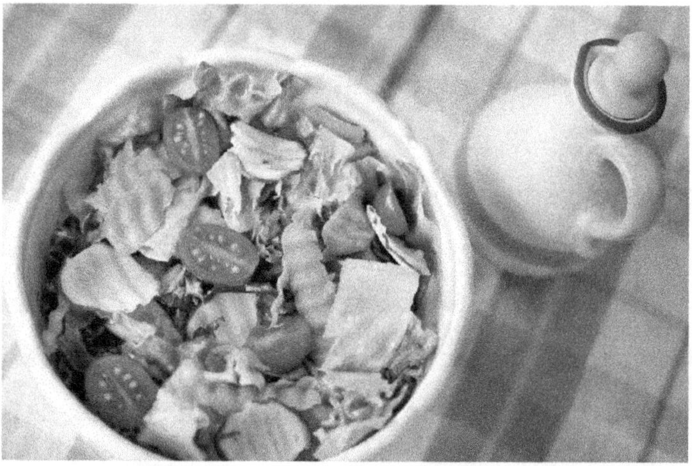

Who says salads are boring? Using green leaf lettuce as a base, you can add all kinds of vegetables, cheese and protein ingredients to make a delicious lunch or dinner with barely any cooking required. Add in bacon and you have something rich in protein, fiber as well as flavor.

Ingredients

6 ounces raw bacon

2 cups green leaf lettuce

4 ounces hard cheese, cut into strips

1 handful cherry tomatoes, halved

3-4 radishes, sliced

1 cucumber, sliced into strips

Freshly ground black pepper to taste

1 tablespoon full-fat dressing, sugar free

1 teaspoon lemon juice (optional)

Steps

Step One: Cooking the Bacon

Cook the bacon in a skillet according to the instructions. Once cooked to your desired crispness, remove from heat pat away the fat with a paper towel. Chop the bacon into bite sized pieces and set aside.

Step Two: Making the Salad

Rip the lettuce into bite sized pieces (you can just use your hands or rough chop with a chef's knife). Chop up the tomatoes, cucumber, radishes and cheese in strips or as you'd like. Toss everything together and add in the bacon. Add in the dressing and lemon juice.

Step Three: Storage

If you're not ready to eat the salad right away, you can store it in a mason jar in layers. Pour the dressing on the bottom, followed by the tomatoes, cucumbers, cheese and lettuce on the top.

Tips

Make this salad into a filling entrée by adding chopped hard boiled eggs, chicken and avocado. If you're looking for a meatless option, try with black beans instead of bacon or chicken. Also try with other types of veggies and cheeses, such as zucchini, mushrooms, feta or Swiss cheese.

Protein Trail Mix

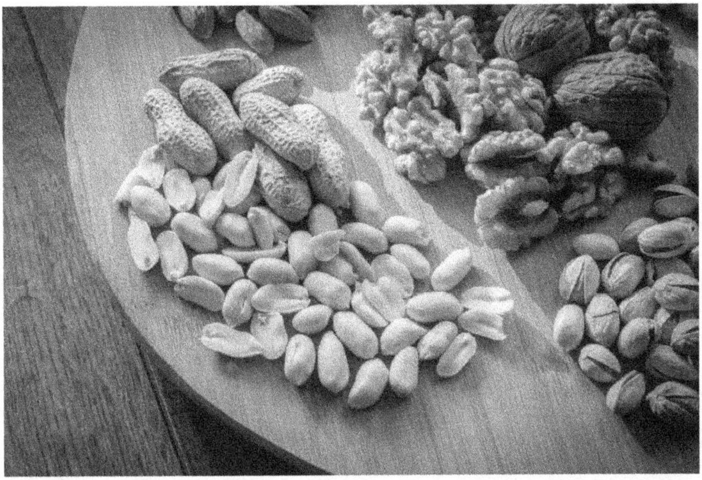

Now that you're in Phase 2 of the Atkins diet, you can start eating more nuts, dried fruit and even chocolate in moderation. One great way to fight mid-morning or afternoon cravings is to have an easy to eat and access snack by your side whenever hunger strikes. Try this homemade trail mix recipe or change it up to suit your tastes.

Ingredients

2 cups mixed nuts

½ cup chocolate candies or unsweetened chocolate chips

½ cup raisins

½ cup seeds

Steps

Step One: Choosing Your Mix

A great trail mix has your favorite types of nuts, whether that be Brazil nuts, almonds, walnuts, peanuts, pecans, hazelnuts and so on. While shopping for nuts, look in the bulk section and buy unsalted so you can control the salt content when you make the mix. Some dried fruit and seed options include pumpkin seeds, sunflower seeds, raisins, dried cranberries and dried blueberries. Avoid buying dried fruit with added sugar and look for natural, unsweetened options. If you'd rather not use chocolate chips, you can use unsweetened coconut instead.

Step Two: Putting it All Together

In a large mixing bowl, pour the nuts, seeds, chocolate chips and dried fruit together and mix using a spoon. If you're looking to add a bit of flavor to pull everything together, you can put in a pinch of nutmeg, half a teaspoon of cinnamon and a pinch of sea salt.

Step Three: Storage

Divide into single serve Ziploc bags and keep with you on car trips, hikes and ball games.

Tips

You can double or triple this recipe as needed. Trail mix can be put together in large portions, so you can save time by making a large batch and storing in containers or distributing into serving size bags.

Buffalo Chicken Wings with Blue Cheese Dipping Sauce

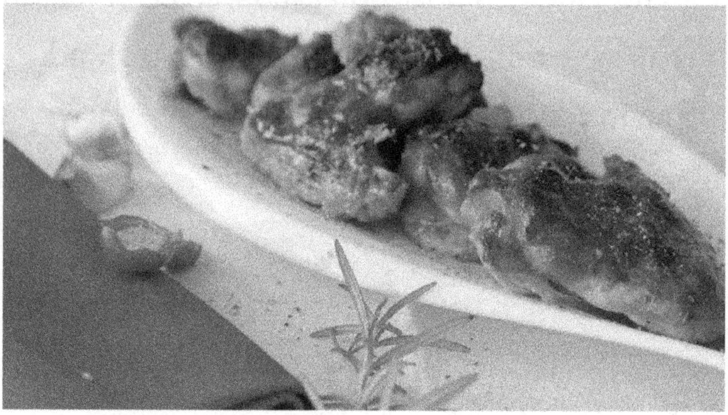

Chicken wings are juicy, full of flavor and you can dress them up to taste like whatever you're in the mood for, from Asian to buffalo style. While chicken wings are usually associated with being a high-calorie fried food, they can also be cooked in a way that transforms them into a delicious and healthy meal.

Ingredients

For the chicken:

2 pounds wings and/or drumsticks

½ teaspoon garlic powder

½ black pepper

1 cup apple cider vinegar

1/8 tablespoon cayenne or red pepper

¼ teaspoon celery salt

For the dipping sauce:

1 cup Greek yogurt (plain unsweetened)

½ cup blue cheese, crumbled (optional)

1 tablespoon lemon juice

Steps

Step One: Marinating the Chicken

In a large mixing bowl, combine the garlic powder, apple cider vinegar, celery salt and cayenne pepper. Toss the chicken in the marinade, cover the bowl with a lid or plastic wrap and set in the fridge for 30 minutes.

Step Two: Cooking the Chicken

Preheat your oven to 375 degrees Fahrenheit. Line the chicken wings and drumsticks evenly on a baking sheet. Reserve some of the marinade for basting. Bake the chicken for 30 minutes. Turn the chicken and baste with wings. Bake for 25 minutes, basting the wings frequently without taking them out of the oven. Once cooked, remove the pan from the oven and allow the chicken wings to cool while sitting in the pan.

Step Three: Serving

While the chicken is cooking, mix together the dipping sauce ingredients and store in the refrigerator until the chicken is ready to eat. Serve the chicken with the blue cheese dip.

Tips

For the dipping sauce, instead of Greek yogurt, you can use ½ cup of sour cream and a cup of mayonnaise instead. If you'd like extra spice, put ¼ cup hot sauce into the marinade (just make sure it has no added sugar).

Beef Sauté with Bell Peppers, Onions and Cheese

If you're looking for a rich, easy and fun weeknight meal, beef sauté is a very convenient and affordable option that the whole family will enjoy eating. Why spend hours in the kitchen when you could be using the time for family or personal enjoyment? This beef sauté recipe can be made all in one skillet, so clean up is a breeze.

Ingredients

1 pound ground beef, 80% lean (you can also use 1 pound beef loin steak, cut into strips)

2 green bell peppers

1 red bell pepper

1 yellow bell pepper

1 large onion

2 garlic cloves

½ cup Cheddar cheese, shredded

¼ teaspoon black pepper

¼ cup olive oil

1 tablespoon low sodium soy sauce

Steps

Step One: Cooking the Beef

If you're using steak strips, pat them dry and stir-fry the steak in a heavy skillet oiled with olive oil and heated to medium-high heat. If you're using ground beef, you should only need a very small amount of cooking oil or none depending on the fat content of the beef (oil isn't needed for beef with higher fat content). Cook the beef until browned and cooked through, 3-4 minutes. If you're using steak strips, transfer to a plate and cover with a paper towel to cool. If you're using ground beef, you can add in the bell peppers, onions and garlic straight away.

Step Two: Cooking the Vegetables

Cook the peppers, onions and garlic with the ground beef on medium-high heat until softened. If you're using steak strips, add in a little bit of olive oil to the pan and cook the bell peppers, onions and garlic by themselves until soft and golden, then add the steak strips back to the pan.

Step Three: Serving

Remove the beef and vegetables from heat and drain any excess fat before serving on a plate.

Sprinkle the cheese on top immediately so it can melt. If you're saving leftovers, allow to cool and store in an airtight container in the refrigerator for 3 to 4 days.

Tips

This recipe pairs well with cooked brown rice (1/2 cup is a serving), but you can also use cauliflower rice if you want to stay as low carb as possible.

Grilled Pork Tenderloin with Cabbage Apple Slaw

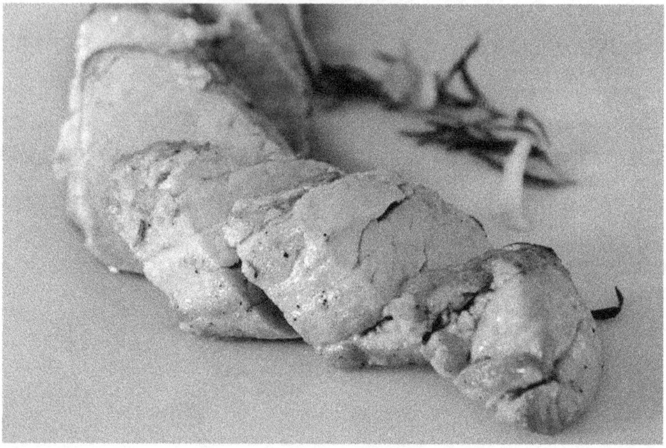

While pork usually isn't associated with health food, it can still be part of a healthy diet if eaten in moderation. Pork tenderloin is an especially lean cut of pork that can be a great source of lean protein with minimal saturated fat.

Ingredients

For the pork:

1 whole pork tenderloin (1-2 pounds)

1 tablespoon olive oil

½ teaspoon garlic powder

½ cup lime juice

Salt and pepper to taste

For the cabbage slaw:

1 tablespoon olive oil

8 cups of red cabbage, shredded

1 whole onion, diced

1 whole apple, cored and sliced (with or without skin)

4 tablespoons red wine vinegar

½ cup water

Steps

Step One: Preparing and Cooking the Pork

Rub the pork tenderloin with salt, pepper, garlic powder and one tablespoon of olive oil. You can also marinate the pork tenderloin in a bag with these ingredients along with some lime juice. Ideally, pork tenderloin should be marinated for 6 to 24 hours. To cook the pork, you can either grill it or use a sauté pan. If you're going to grill it, place it on a cooking grate heated to medium-high. Cook on one side for about 5 minutes, then roll the tenderloin over and grill the other side for 5 minutes. Do the same for the rest of the sides until the whole tenderloin has a nice brown crust. You'll know it's done when the internal temperature reads 150 degrees. Remove the tenderloin from the grill and cover with tin foil for about 10 minutes. Do not slice into it until you let it rest. Alternatively, you can sauté the tenderloin in a skillet with oil over medium heat for 5 or 6 minutes, then place it in the oven on a baking sheet at 425 degrees and cook until down, which should be in 15 to 20 minutes. Again, the meat needs to rest.

Step Two: Cooking the Cabbage

In a large skillet, heat a tablespoon of olive oil and stir in the chopped onions and cabbage. Cook the onions on medium heat for 1 or 2 minutes until translucent and then add in the cabbage. Cook for another minute or two and then add in the apples, vinegar, water, salt and pepper. Simmer for 10 minutes covered, and another 10 minutes uncovered. The slaw will need to be stirred occasionally.

Step Three: Serving

Once rested, cut the pork tenderloin by slicing diagonally and serve with the cabbage slaw. If you prefer to have your slaw taste a little sweeter, you can add 2 tablespoons of a sugar substitute during the cooking process.

Tips

When marinating pork tenderloin, you can experiment with a variety of flavors and seasonings. For example, you can try ginger and soy sauce or balsamic vinegar and garlic.

Cauliflower Pizza with Tomato and Bacon

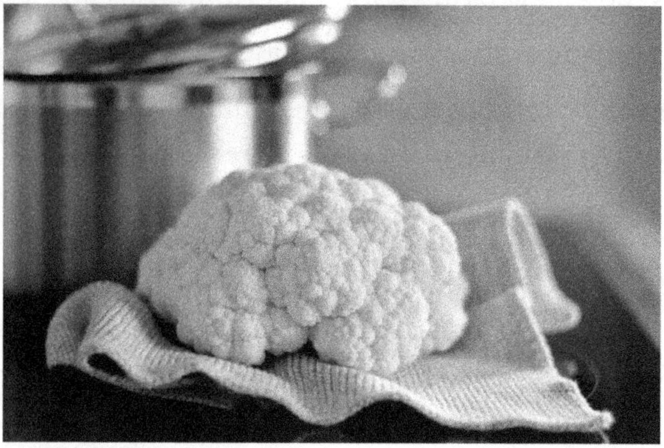

It might be time to change up your Saturday night pizza party with this delicious and unique recipe that uses cauliflower instead of pizza dough. It still tastes crispy, cheesy and garlicy, yet it has much less carbs and calories than traditional style pizza. Give it a try – you just might have a new favorite!

Ingredients

1 head cauliflower

½ cup shredded mozzarella, plus extra for topping

2 whole eggs

¼ cup Parmesan, grated

1 teaspoon dried oregano

1 teaspoon fresh parsley

¼ teaspoon garlic powder

1 tomato, cut into slices

¼ cup cooked bacon, chopped into pieces

Steps

Step One: Prepare the Cauliflower

Make sure the cauliflower is washed and patted dry. Cut the cauliflower into florets and remove the stalk. You can either use a cheese grater or a food processor to make the cauliflower crust. In a food processor, pulse the cauliflower florets until they have a fine texture. For cooking, you can either steam them in a steamer basket on the strove for 5 minutes or cook them covered in a microwave for 8 minutes. Allow the cauliflower to cool and then drain them as best you can by pressing the water out with a towel.

Step Two: Making the Pizza

Preheat your oven to 400 degrees Fahrenheit. Whisk the eggs until combined. In a large bowl, mix the eggs with the cauliflower along with the mozzarella, Parmesan, oregano and garlic powder. Get out a pan or baking sheet and press the mixture evenly onto the sheet so it resembles a pizza crust. Bake for 15 to 20 minutes until lightly golden.

Step Three: Toppings and Serving

Once cooked, remove the crust from the oven and add the toppings of your choice. Sprinkle your desired amount of mozzarella cheese (or other kind of cheese) along with the tomatoes and bacon. Place back in the oven on high heat and allow the cheese to melt, up to 10 minutes. Serve hot.

Tips

If you want the pizza to have a more traditional taste, you can spread unsweetened tomato sauce on the crust before putting on your toppings. You can also experiment with different low-carb sauces and toppings, such as garlic paste, pesto or salsa.

Dessert

Coconut Cookies

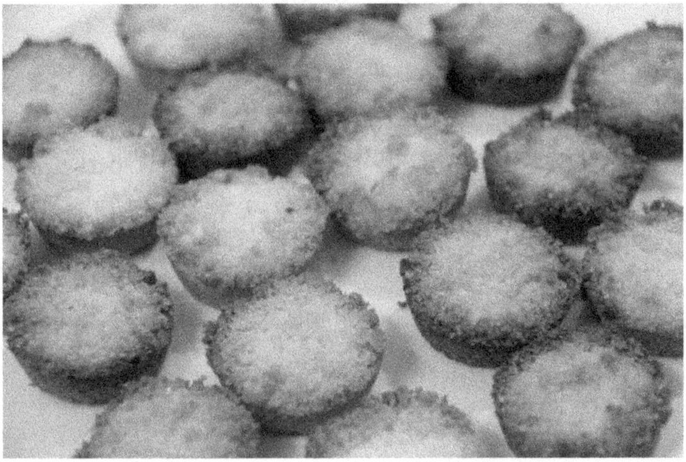

Cookies can be a guilty pleasure, but they don't always have to be chocked full of carbs. This coconut cook recipe uses "unsweetened" flavors and healthier flour alternatives while still producing a tasty dessert.

Ingredients

1/3 cup dried coconut

5 tablespoons unsweetened coconut milk

1 tablespoon vanilla extract

1 tablespoon coconut extract (optional)

½ teaspoon salt

½ cup unsweetened shredded coconut

1 cup almond flour or whole grain soy flour

Steps

Step One: Making the Batter

In a large mixing bowl, whisk the coconut milk, vanilla, coconut extract and salt until the mixture reaches a smooth consistency. Stir in the almond flour or soy flour and the dried coconut. For best results, cover the dough and let it chill in the fridge for 5 minutes.

Step Two: Baking the Cookies

Using a spoon, scoop the dough and drop onto a baking sheet that's been sprayed with cooking spray. Make sure each scoop is about one tablespoon in size. The balls should be 1 or 2 inches apart. Bake the cookies for 14 to 20 minutes or until golden brown.

Step Three: Storage

Allow the cookies to cool on a tray before serving. Store in parchment paper for up to 5 days in the fridge.

Tips

If the cookies aren't sweet enough for you, you can add in a tablespoon or so of sugar substitute into the batter. Instead of coconut milk, you can also use two egg whites and 8 tablespoons of butter instead (textures will vary).

Chapter Four: Phase 3 Tips and Recipes

Making Dietary Adjustments to Help You Succeed

Phase 3 of the Atkins diet is known as the "pre-maintenance" stage because you should be well on your way to finding the perfect carb balance for your unique lifestyle. This can be an experimental stage where you're going to have a lot of trial and error before moving on to Phase 4. During Phase 3, spend some time finding something that works for you by listening and paying attention to your body and any changes that occur.

You should be close to your goal weight, so determine your actions based on your progress. If you find that you're starting to gain again, you should decrease your carb intake by a certain increment and adjust as needed. If you're continuing to lose weight or you're maintaining a weight that you're happy with, you can move on to Phase 4.

Phase 3 recipes for the Atkins diet will consist of a very balanced meal plan full of proteins, vegetables and some fruits. In this phase, you can start drinking more berry smoothies and using more fruits in recipes, as long as you stick with fresh, wholesome ingredients.

Breakfast

Mixed Berry Parfait

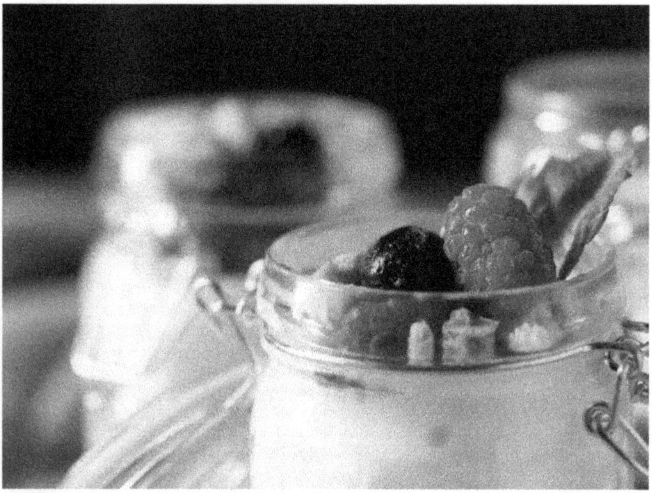

If you love sweet breakfasts, you're in for a treat with this mixed berry parfait that you can have for breakfast, brunch, dessert… whenever you're in the mood!

Ingredients

½ cup Greek yogurt, unsweetened

½ cup heavy cream

1 tablespoon chia seeds

1/3 cup fresh raspberries or berries of your choice

1/3 cup frozen berries

1 tablespoon honey or maple syrup

¼ cup sliced almonds

¼ dried coconut

1 tablespoon flax seeds

Steps

Step One: Making the Granola

Pre-heat your oven to 350 degrees Fahrenheit. On a baking sheet, spread out the nuts, seeds and coconut. Toss in the honey or maple syrup and distribute evenly to make the granola mixture. Bake in the oven for 20 to 30 minutes until crunchy and golden. You may need to stir every ten minutes or so to ensure the mixtures. Set granola aside and allow to cool.

Step Two: Preparing the Berries and Yogurt

Blend the frozen berries in a blender until smooth. Clean and pat dry the fresh berries. You can use only fresh berries or only frozen berries depending on your preference. In a small bowl, mix together the Greek yogurt, heavy cream and chia seeds. Place in the fridge until you're ready to eat.

Step Three: Layering and Serving

Get out four glasses (or as needed) and distribute the parfait in layers. Start by adding a scoop of the yogurt mixture followed by the frozen berry puree. Add a scoop of the granola and then put on another layer of the yogurt mixture. Top with more granola and fresh berries. Enjoy cold.

Tips

There's several different ways you can make granola, and making it at home is a great way to control the sugar and salt content. Experiment with different flavor combinations and store granola in containers for up to two months.

Cinnamon Waffles

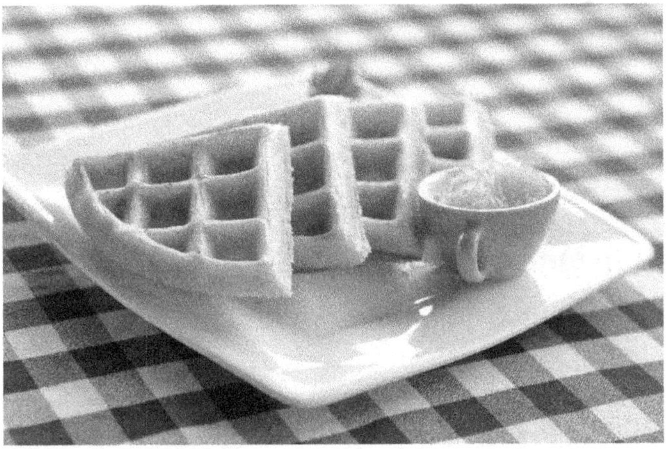

Waffles are always a favorite, but many people try to avoid them because they're often overloaded with carbs. Luckily, there's a few ways to make healthy waffles that still taste scrumptious while remaining fairly low in carbs. Try opting for whole grain or almond based flours and use natural fruit as a topping.

Ingredients

2 whole egg yolks

1 teaspoon vanilla extract

1 cup whole buttermilk

¼ cup butter (melted)

1 cup almond flour or whole grain soy flour

1 ½ teaspoons baking powder

½ teaspoon baking soda

½ tablespoon sugar substitute

¼ teaspoon salt

½ tablespoon cinnamon

Steps

Step One: Making the Batter

In a medium bowl, whisk together the eggs with the vanilla, buttermilk and melted butter. Make sure the mixture is well-blended, and then add the almond or whole grain soy flour, baking soda, baking powder, sugar substitute, salt and cinnamon. Stir everything together thoroughly.

Step Two: Making the Waffles

Preheat your waffle iron on its normal setting. Spoon in the batter and fill appropriately. Close the waffle iron and cook the waffles until golden brown to your liking. Continue with the rest of the batter.

Step Three: Serving

Serve hot waffles immediately and top with a dollop of Greek yogurt or heavy cream and ½ cup of fresh fruit. You can freeze leftover waffles for 3 to 4 months – just microwave or put in a toaster when you're ready to eat them.

Tips

If you want fluffier waffles, you can first separate the yolks and whites from the two eggs. Whisk the egg whites with an electric mixture until they form stiff peaks, then fold into the waffle batter.

Spicy Veggie Egg Breakfast Burrito

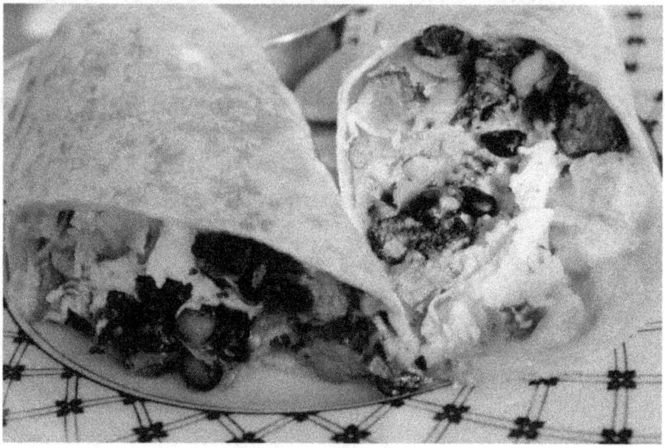

Breakfast burritos are really the ultimate breakfast foods because you can fill them with whatever ingredients you want and take them with you without worrying about very much cleanup. While this recipe doesn't include meat, you can fill your burrito up with bacon, turkey sausage or tofu if you're looking for extra energy and protein.

Ingredients

2 whole wheat tortillas (look for low carb options)

4 eggs

1 tablespoon olive oil or coconut oil

1/8 teaspoon red or cayenne pepper

1 jalapeno

1 red bell pepper

½ cup shredded cheddar cheese

2 ounces spicy salsa

Steps

Step One: Starting the Vegetables

If you'd like to brown your tortilla, use a skillet to warm them on both sides on medium heat for about one minute and then set aside. Slice the jalapeno and bell pepper into strips or bite sized pieces. Put the oil in a skillet and heat to medium, then add the bell pepper and jalapeno. Cook until softened, for about three minutes.

Step Two: Cooking the Eggs

In a small bowl, whisk the eggs together and add in the cayenne pepper. You can also add black pepper if you'd like. Pour the eggs into the skillet with the peppers and stir them until they begin to set. This should only take about two minutes.

Step Three: Serving

When the eggs are cooked, remove the skillet from the burner and divide the egg mixture into the tortillas evenly. Sprinkle in the cheese. You can either spread salsa on top or have salsa on the side as dipping sauce. Roll the tortillas up gently to form burritos.

Tips

Breakfast burritos are also great with onions, mushrooms, cheese, avocado and more. Make a batch ahead and wrap them up individual. Keep them in the fridge for 3 to 4 days and grab them in the morning or whenever you need a quick meal.

Lunch and Snacks

Cheeseburger Stuffed Peppers

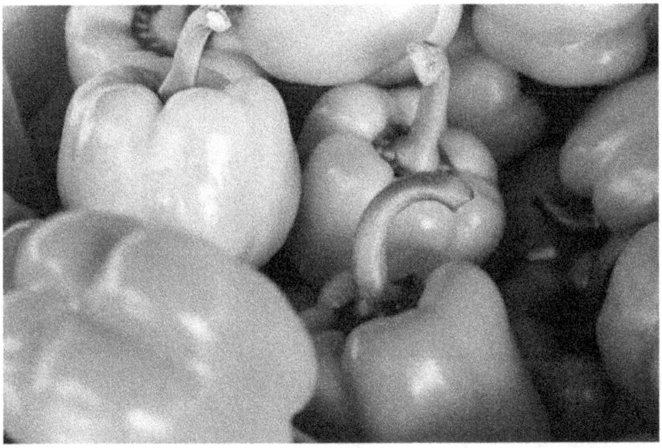

Bell peppers are the secret superheroes of the vegetable world. They're extremely versatile and they come in a variety of different colors and flavors. Stuffed peppers is a delicious and easy way to have a filling meal without the need to add carb-loaded buns or bread. Next time you're craving a cheese burger or something cheesy and meaty, try this stuffed pepper recipe!

Ingredients

½ pound lean ground beef or turkey

4 large bell peppers

6 ounces cheddar cheese, shredded

½ red onion, diced

Salt and pepper to taste

Avocado for topping (optional)

1 tablespoon olive oil

Steps

Step One: Preparing the Peppers

Clean the bell peppers and pat dry. Cut them in half, lengthwise, and remove all the stems, ribs and seeds from inside. Be careful not to rip them open – you want to them hold in the stuffing while cooking.

Step Two: Making the Filling

In a medium skillet, cook the ground beef on medium-high until browned and cooked through. Make sure to season with salt and pepper. Add in the onion and cook until soft and caramelized. Add in the cheese and then start stuffing the peppers with the filling.

Step Three: Baking

Preheat your oven to 400 degrees Fahrenheit. Set the stuffed peppers in a baking dish and drizzle them with the olive oil. Cover the bell peppers with aluminum foil and bake them for 30 minutes. Check them and remove the foil, then bake for another 15 minutes. You want the cheese to get golden brown. Serve warm or let cool and store in the fridge for 3 to 4 days.

Tips

Try different stuffing combinations depending on what you're in the mood for. You can also exclude the meat complete for a vegetarian option. Craving pizza? Try peppers stuffed with feta cheese, mozzarella cheese, tomatoes and basil.

Peanut Chicken Skewers

Are you looking for a light and delicious lunch or meal that you can have at parties to impress your guests or kids? Make these fun chicken skewers or change them up with any kind of meat or vegetable you'd like.

Ingredients

2 cooked chicken breasts, cut into strips

½ small onion

3 teaspoons garlic powder

4 teaspoons curry powder

1 teaspoon cumin

1 teaspoon ground ginger

½ teaspoon red or cayenne pepper

1 cup heavy cream

1/3 cup low sodium, natural creamy peanut butter

1 lime

1/3 cup water

Salt and pepper to taste

Steps

Step One: Marinating and Skewering the Chicken

Before using the skewers, make sure to soak them for at least 20 minutes or overnight so they don't burn while grilling. In a blender or food processor, blend together the cream, onion, garlic powder, curry powder, cumin, cayenne and ginger. Add salt and pepper as needed (or make sure the chicken is already seasoned). Make sure you get a smooth consistency. Toss the cooked chicken in the marinade and let it sit at room temperature for about 15 minutes.

Step Two: Making the Sauce

In a blender or food processor, mix together the peanut butter, water and all the juice from the lime. You can also add in a couple cloves of garlic if you want extra flavor. Blend until smooth and transfer to a small bowl or container that you can cover and refrigerate until serving time.

Step Three: Cooking the Skewers

Turn on your broiler or grill. Skewer the marinated chicken pieces and place them on an oiled rack where they cannot fall through. Cook them for about 5 minutes, turning once, to ensure even doneness. Serve with the peanut dipping sauce.

Tips

Try this recipe with beef skewers or shrimp skewers. You can also change up the sauce and marinade to your liking. If you want the sauce to be sweeter, add in two teaspoons of sugar substitute.

Butternut Squash Soup with Sour Cream

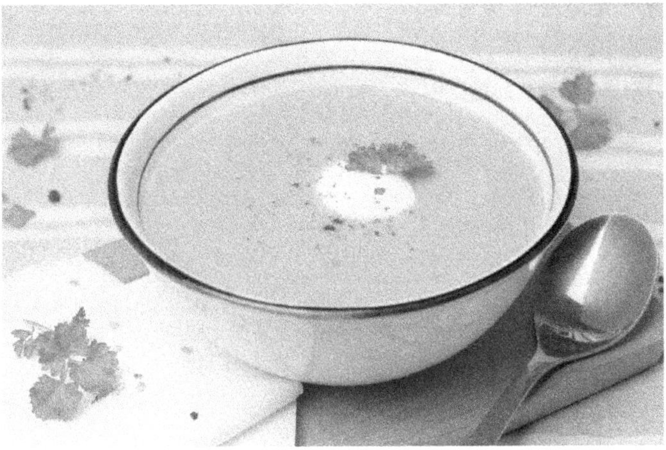

Ingredients

1 medium butternut squash

1 cup heavy cream

1 cup chicken broth or stock

1 sweet onion

Salt and pepper to taste

½ teaspoon nutmeg

½ teaspoon garlic salt

2 tablespoons olive oil

Steps

Step One: Preparing the Squash

Prepare the squash by cutting the top and bottom off so you can stabilize it on the counter. Carefully use a sharp knife to cut the skin away on all sides. Cut the squash in half and take out the seeds. After peeling, cut the squash into cubes.

Step Two: Roasting the Squash

Preheat your oven to 450 degrees Fahrenheit. Get out a baking sheet and distribute the squash cubes on the sheet. Toss the cubes with a tablespoon of olive oil and add salt and pepper. Roast them in the oven for 30 or 40 minutes or until tender, turning once or twice.

Step Three: Making the Soup

In a large pot, cook the onions until soft and fragrant. Once you've removed the roasted squash from the oven, transfer to the pot with the onions. Put the pot on medium heat and add in the broth, nutmeg and garlic salt, then bring to a boil. Let the mixture simmer on low heat for about 20 minutes after it starts to boil. After 20 minutes, stir in the heavy cream and add any more spices as desired. Use an immersion blender or a regular blender to puree the soup into a smooth and creamy texture. Add in more pepper as needed.

Tips

Serve the soup hot with a dollop of sour cream. You can also top it with toasted squash or pumpkin seeds. Store the leftovers in a container and freeze for up to 3 months.

Foil Packet Fish and Vegetables

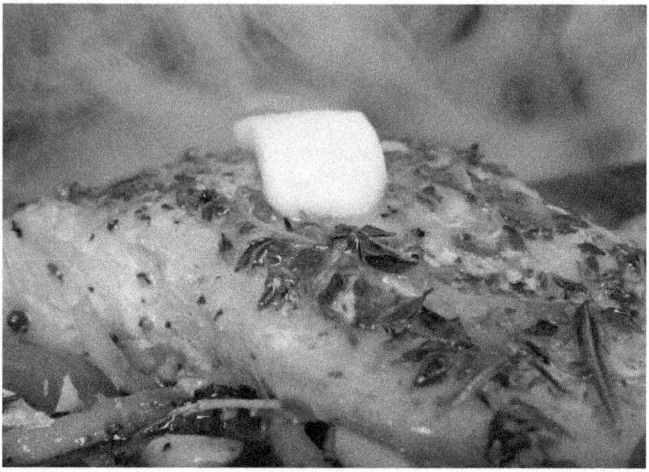

If you're not used to cooking fish, you may be worried about drying it out or undercooking it. You might also be worried about making a mess, but there's no need to stress with this convenient foil fish recipe. By cooking fish in a foil, you can also add in vegetables and seasonings and have everything done and ready to go at one time.

Ingredients

A fish of your choice, such as four 6 ounce salmon fillets or 1 ½ pounds large shrimp

4 cups of two or three vegetables of your choice, such as 1 cup sliced onion, 2 cups sliced zucchini and 1 cup cherry tomatoes

2 garlic cloves

½ cup lemon juice

2 tablespoons olive oil

Your choice of herbs, including parsley, rosemary, oregano or thyme.

Salt and pepper to taste

Steps

Step One: Putting Together the Foil Pack

Get out a large sheet of tin foil for each fish fillet you have. In each foil, start by laying down an even amount of vegetables and then adding in the seasonings and herbs of your choice. Set the fish fillet on top of the vegetables (you can do this the other way around if you prefer) and drizzle with olive oil and lemon juice. You can also use water, balsamic vinegar or white wine depending on your flavor preferences.

Step Two: Cooking

Preheat your oven to 450 degrees Fahrenheit. Once you've compiled your packet of fish and vegetables, wrap up the tin foil and fold on all sides so that everything holds tightly together. Now, you can either cook the fish in the oven or on a grill or campfire. To cook in the oven, bake for 12 to 20 minutes (more vegetables and larger fillets should be cooked longer). You want to make sure the fish gets cooked through. If you need to check, lift up one corner and carefully poke the fish with a fork to see if it flakes. Once you take the packet out of the oven, don't open right away – allow the packet to sit for about 5 minutes.

Step Three: Serving

Fish and vegetable packets can be eaten as is or topped with your choice of a low-carb topping. Try melting together freshly squeezed lemon with a little bit of butter and a pinch of ground ginger.

Tips

The great thing about this recipe is that you can change it up whenever you feel like it or modify it according to what ingredients are in season. You can also prepare the ingredients ahead of time to take with you on a camping trip. To cook in a campfire, place it on a cooking grate and cook for 10 to 12 minutes and let sit an additional 5 minutes.

1 lemon

¼ ounce cilantro (leaves only)

¼ cup chopped fresh parsley (leaves only)

2 ½ tablespoons olive oil

Salt and pepper to taste

For the cauliflower:

1 head cauliflower

2 cups water

1 tablespoon sour cream

1 tablespoon butter (unsalted)

Salt and pepper to taste

Steps

Step One: Making the Topping

In a food processor, blend together the cilantro, parsley, shallot, half of the juice from the lemon, garlic clove, red wine vinegar, and pepper. Pulse the ingredients (you can also mix them by hand in a bowl if you need to) so that they're well combined (they shouldn't be heavily pureed). Finally, add in two tablespoons of olive oil and mix well. Set aside in a medium bowl.

Step Two: Making the Cauliflower

Cut the stem from the cauliflower and chop it into florets. Steam the cauliflower in a steamer

1 lemon

¼ ounce cilantro (leaves only)

¼ cup chopped fresh parsley (leaves only)

2 ½ tablespoons olive oil

Salt and pepper to taste

For the cauliflower:

1 head cauliflower

2 cups water

1 tablespoon sour cream

1 tablespoon butter (unsalted)

Salt and pepper to taste

Steps

Step One: Making the Topping

In a food processor, blend together the cilantro, parsley, shallot, half of the juice from the lemon, garlic clove, red wine vinegar, and pepper. Pulse the ingredients (you can also mix them by hand in a bowl if you need to) so that they're well combined (they shouldn't be heavily pureed). Finally, add in two tablespoons of olive oil and mix well. Set aside in a medium bowl.

Step Two: Making the Cauliflower

Cut the stem from the cauliflower and chop it into florets. Steam the cauliflower in a steamer

Seared Steak with Mashed Cauliflower

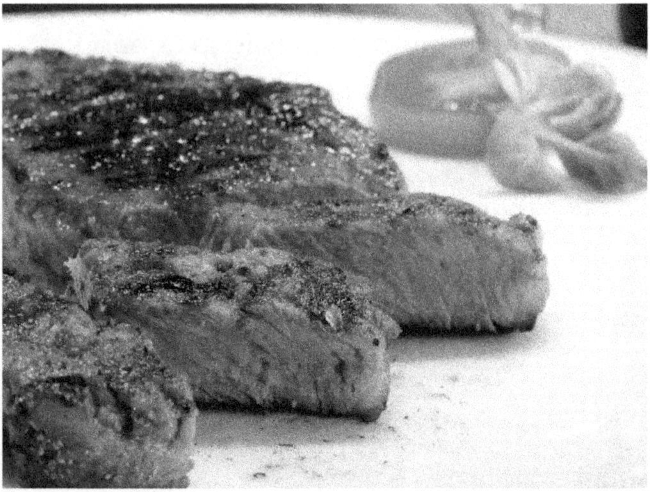

There's nothing like a steak and potato dinner, but white potatoes should generally be excluded while living on a low-carb diet. What to do? Cauliflower is your answer! Cauliflower can be cooked and doctored up to have a similar taste and feel as mashed potatoes with much less carbs, and it also tastes great with a nice cut of lean steak.

Ingredients

For the steak and topping:

2 strip steaks (about 1 inch thick)

1 shallot, diced

1 garlic clove

1 tablespoon red wine vinegar

basket with two cups of water. The water should be on high heat. Let it come to a boil and cook the cauliflower for 10 to 12 minutes until soft and tender. Drain the cauliflower and then transfer it to a bowl or food processor (if you're using the same food processor as the first step, make sure it's cleaned out). Add in the sour cream, butter, salt and pepper to the food processor and puree with the cauliflower until it reaches a smooth consistency (if you don't want to use butter, you can use 2 tablespoons olive oil instead).

Step Three: Cooking the Steak

In a large skillet, heat the last ½ tablespoon of olive oil on medium-high heat. Season the steaks with salt and pepper and then place into the hot pan. For a medium-rare steak, cook 4 to 5 minutes on all sides. Allow the steak at least 5 to 10 minutes to rest before serving. When you're ready to serve, put one steak on a plate with half the cauliflower puree and drizzle on the topping.

Tips

If you'd like to spice this up, add in crushed red pepper chili flakes and cayenne pepper to the topping mixture.

Chicken Cheese Stuffed Quesadillas

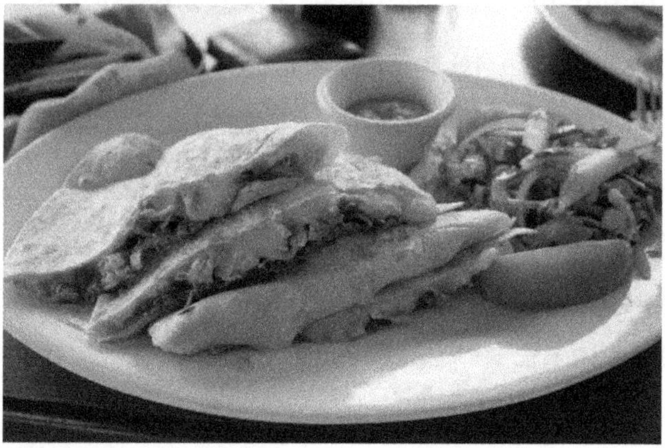

Quesadillas are a fast and fun weeknight dinner idea that can also be modified into a healthy and affordable meal for the whole family. No matter what kind of protein you're in the mood for, you can add it into this flavorful recipe for cheesy stuffed quesadillas.

Ingredients

Your choice of protein, such as 4 cooked 3-ounce chicken breasts, shredded

2-3 bell peppers, cooked (roasted or sautéed)

3 scallions, medium

1/3 cup cilantro (leaves only)

1 cup Monterey jack cheese, shredded

8 whole wheat or low carb tortillas

3 tablespoons butter (unsalted)

Steps

Step One: Preparing the Stuffing

Shred the cooked chicken and dice the bell peppers into bite sized pieces. Dice up the scallions as well. Take four of the tortillas and lay them out on a flat surface. Take ½ cup of the cheese and spread evenly across the tortillas, then lay down an even amount of chicken on all the tortillas. Top with the peppers and scallions (if you'd like you can also put in jalapeno and sautéed onion). Sprinkle on chopped cilantro leaves and the rest of the cheese so that there's enough to melt on both sides. Lastly, set the remaining four tortillas on top of the filled ones.

Step Two: Cooking the Quesadillas

You can either use one large flat griddle or two large skillets (or work in batches). Heat butter on nonstick skillets over medium-high heat. Make sure the butter gets completely melted. Unless you're using mini tortillas or a very large griddle, there should only be one tortilla per skillet. Place the quesadilla carefully on the skillet and cook for about 2 or three minutes. Using a wide spatula, carefully flip the tortilla and cook for another 2 or 3 minutes.

Cook all of the remaining tortillas in the same way. Alternatively, you can brush the tortillas with olive oil on both of the outer sides and cook in the oven on a baking sheet for about 5 minutes at 450 degrees Fahrenheit. When done, they should be crispy, golden and the cheese should be melted.

Step Three: Serving

Tortillas will most easily be eaten if cut into wedges. You have a wide range of options for toppings, including avocado, sour cream, salsa, jalapeno pieces or bell pepper strips. If you'd like to have these quesadillas with guacamole, you can simply mash together half an avocado with 1/3 cup salsa, two tablespoons sour cream, a squirt of lime juice, salt and pepper.

Tips

Try these quesadillas with strips of steak, shredded beef, black beans or tofu strips for something unique to your tastes. This is a somewhat higher-carb meal, so limit to one or two days a week or as needed according to your dietary needs.

Dessert

Berries and Cream

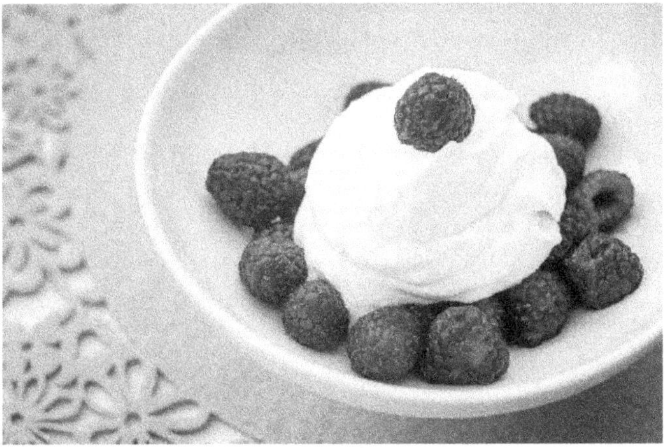

If you're looking for something light and fruity yet decadent and low-carb, fresh berries with your choice of cream is a great dessert that will surely satisfy your sweet tooth. This dessert is light, easy and you can enjoy it in moderation any time of day when you want something sweet and rich.

Ingredients

1/2 cup raspberries

1/2 cup blueberries

1/3 cup heavy cream or Greek yogurt (unsweetened)

1 tablespoon vanilla extract

1 teaspoon lemon zest (optional)

1 teaspoon cinnamon (optional)

1 teaspoon almonds or crushed nuts (optional)

Steps

Step One: Preparing the Berries

Thoroughly rinse the fresh berries and pat dry. You can also use frozen berries or a mixture of fresh and frozen.

Step Two: Making the Cream

Depending on your preference and what you have on hand, you can use heavy cream, Greek yogurt or coconut cream as the base to go with the fruit. You can even use combinations, just be mindful of carb intake. In a medium bowl, whip together the heavy cream with the vanilla extract and add in any other flavors you'd like, such as lemon zest or cinnamon.

Step Three: Serving

In a small bowl, ramekin, dessert cup or martini glass (depending on how fancy you want to be), drop in the cream mixture and top with the fresh berries. If you'd like you can also use strawberries, sliced peaches, pomegranate seeds or any other fruit and berries that are in season.

Tips

You can experiment with this dessert by adding your own unique topping choices, such as crushed nuts, homemade granola, shredded coconut or sweet spices. If you don't want to use vanilla extract, you can use 1-2 tablespoons of a sugar substitute or ½ tablespoon honey.

Chapter Five: Phase 4 Tips and Recipes

Striking a Balance to Last a Lifetime

Phase 4 is arguably the most important phase of the Atkins diet. It's no longer a diet but a lifestyle to be maintained, adapted and celebrated. Food is a huge part of our lives, and that's why having a great, healthy relationship with food is essential for a more balanced, fulfilling lifestyle. Phase 4 is the maintenance phase where you start using Atkins diet tools and concepts to continuing losing weight or maintain your happy weight for the rest of your life.

During phase 4, you can start incorporating some other types of healthy carbs aside from fruits and vegetables, such as oats, brown rice, sweet potato and quinoa. These carbs should still be eaten in moderation. At this point, you should have a better understanding of your body and how it responds to changes in your diet. You should know the basics of carb balance, especially in terms of how to keep your weight down by living on a lower carb diet even after you've reached your goal weight. It is okay if you have to back-peddle to one of the previous stages – as long as you keep putting in the effort, you will see results.

Breakfast

Creamy Oatmeal with Fruit

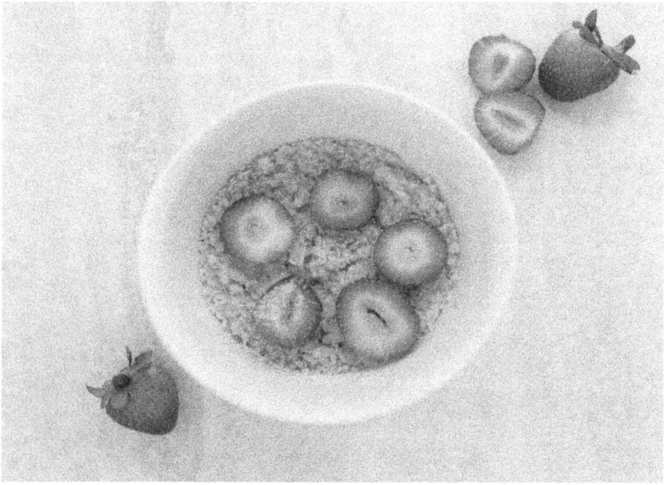

Oats and oatmeal can be party of any healthy diet, as long as you opt for raw, unsweetened oats that have no added sugar or flavorings. The fun thing about buying plain oatmeal is that you can add in the flavors you want while also controlling how much sugar goes into your breakfast! While oatmeal does contain carbs, old fashioned, unsweetened oatmeal is full of fiber and can help you feel satisfied for longer, making it a great addition to any weight loss diet (however, oatmeal should be excluded during the first 2 phases of the Atkins diet).

Ingredients

¼ cup rolled oats, uncooked (preferably Gluten Free)

½ cup water

¼ chopped nuts of your choice, such as pecans

1/4 cup sliced fruit or berries of your choice

1 tablespoon heavy cream or Greek yogurt, unsweetened (optional)

Steps

Step One: Making the Oats

Cook oats according to the instructions. Usually, rolled oats or old fashion oats are made by mixing the water with the oats and cooking on high in the microwave for about 2 to 3 minutes, stirring before serving. If you'd like to use a stovetop, bring water to a boil in a pot with a pinch of salt and add in the oats. Bring the heat from high down to a simmer and cook for about 5 minutes, uncovered, stirring occasionally.

Step Two: Preparing the Toppings

You can use any low-carb, natural toppings you'd like. Sprinkle on some berries and a little bit of crushed nuts, but avoid adding sweeteners as much as possible. You can even use oatmeal and turn it into a savory breakfast by adding mushrooms, onions, tomatoes and other vegetables drizzled with vinegar, lemon juice and spices.

Step Three: Serving the Oatmeal

Stir in the creamy element of your choice and serve with the toppings while the oatmeal is still warm. You can also make overnight oats by mixing raw oats with a thickener such as milk or yogurt and adding fresh toppings when you're ready to eat in the morning.

Tips

Oats are very adaptable and they can be used to replace flour in some baking recipes. You can also put oats in your granola mixture or make oat granola bars. Avoid eating oats in the first two phases of the Atkins diet because oatmeal, like other carb-based foods, may interfere with your weight loss (an exception would be if you are an extremely active person).

Chocolate Protein Shake

Chocolate for breakfast? What more could anyone want? When healthy, natural ingredients are used, chocolate can become a part of your morning routine. This chocolate protein shake will not only help satisfy your sweet tooth but also give you a boost of energy to help power you through a workout or the mid-morning blues.

Ingredients

1 cup coconut milk, unsweetened

1 scoop chocolate protein (whey)

1 tablespoon cocoa powder, unsweetened

2 tablespoons less sodium creamy peanut butter, natural (optional)

¼ teaspoon cinnamon (optional)

½ teaspoon peppermint extract (optional)

½ tablespoon stevia or sugar substitute (optional)

Steps

Step One: Choosing Your Chocolate Base

There are two main sources of low-carb chocolate that you can use as a basis for your chocolate shakes: chocolate whey protein and unsweetened cocoa powder. Use about one scoop of each. Add in a creamy component, either 1 cup of coconut milk, 1 cup of almond milk or 1 cup of soy milk. This will had a creamy richness to the shake.

Step Two: Choosing Your Flavorings

This is where you can start to have fun by trying different flavor combinations that will sweeten up your chocolate shake without adding too much sugar. Try peanut butter with cinnamon or mint extract with ½ cup chopped strawberries (you can also use fresh mint leaves).

Step Three: Blending and Serving

Place all the ingredients in a blender and blend until smooth.

Tips

If you want your chocolate shake cold, add in a few ice cubes. If it's too frothy for your liking, try adding about 3 tablespoons of chia seeds or plain cottage cheese as a thickener.

Spicy Chorizo Frittata

What in the world is a frittata? It's actually a dish made from beaten eggs that have been fried, with an Italian origin. It almost looks like a pizza made of eggs, but you can actually add in all kinds of ingredients to make a unique and flavorful breakfast that will keep you full and satisfied.

Ingredients

6 ounces chorizo

8 whole eggs (large)

2/3 cups chopped red tomatoes or cherry tomatoes

¼ teaspoon crushed red pepper flakes

4 ounces goat or feta cheese (you can also use cheddar cheese)

2 tablespoons basil

Steps

Step One: Preparing the Chorizo

Chorizo is a type of pork sausage full of flavorful spices that you can usually find in the cured meat section at the grocery store. To prepare the chorizo, all you have to do is sauté it over medium-high heat in a large skillet for about 5 minutes. While it's cooking, use a spatula to break up the chorizo into bite-sized pieces. If necessary, drain off excess fat and leave in the pan (the pan will be going in the oven so make sure it's oven-proof).

Step Two: Preparing the Eggs, Tomatoes and Cheese

In a large bowl, lightly beat the eggs and then pour into the pan with the chorizo. Add in the cheese (put some aside for topping if desired), tomatoes, basil and red pepper flakes. You'll need to cook the eggs in the skillet on the stove for about 5 minutes on medium high.

Step Three: Broiling the Frittata

Transfer the eggs and chorizo into your oven preheated to broil. Cook for another 2 to 4 minutes. The frittata should get slightly puffy and set, but not browned. Sprinkle on remaining cheese and serve warm.

Tips

For this recipe, you can also use turkey sausage, cooked ham, mushrooms or any other kind of protein or vegetable of your choice.

Lunch and Snacks

Spiced Zucchini Bread

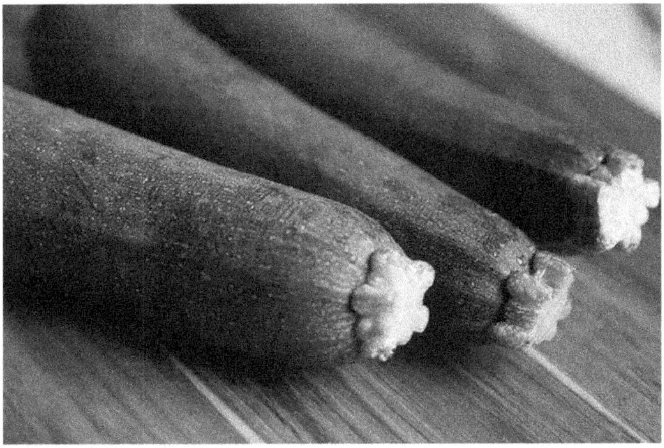

While following a low-carb diet, bread is something you generally want to avoid, even in the later phases of the diet. However, there are some exceptions, especially for homemade breads that are made with high-fiber, low-carb ingredients, such as zucchini bread. Don't be fooled, this bread will taste as good as banana bread and you can have a slice as a lunch or snack.

Ingredients

1 zucchini, large

2 whole eggs (large)

1/3 cup canola vegetable oil

1 teaspoon vanilla extract

½ teaspoon baking soda

½ teaspoon baking powder

1 ½ cups whole wheat pastry flour or flaxseed meal

1/3 cup sugar substitute

1/8 teaspoon nutmeg

1/8 teaspoon allspice

½ teaspoon salt

1 teaspoon ground cinnamon

½ cup walnuts or pecans, roughly chopped and toasted (optional)

Steps

Step One: Making the Batter

Get out three bowls. Using a sharp grater, coarsely grate the zucchini into the first bowl and squeeze out as much excess liquid as you can. In another bowl, mix together the whole wheat flour, baking powder, baking soda, cinnamon, allspice, nutmeg and salt. In the third bowl, use an electric mixer to blend together the sugar substitute, oil, eggs and vanilla. Add the flour mixture from the second bowl into the third bowl with the egg mixture and continue beating on medium speed until well-combined. Finally, add in the zucchini and nuts (if using), and mix well with a spoon.

Step Two: Baking

Preheat your oven to 350 degrees Fahrenheit. Pour the batter into a loaf pan and bake for 50 to 55 minutes or until golden and cooked through. You want to be able to stick a toothpick in and have it come out clean.

Step Three: Serving

Set the loaf pan on a wire cooling rack and allow to cool for 15 to 20 minutes. Serve warm with a small dollop of cream cheese or enjoy plain. Cover the zucchini bread in plastic wrap or foil and keep in the fridge for up to 1 week.

Tips

Use this recipe to make muffins that you can take with you or send with your kids to school in their lunch box. Just use the same batter and pour into cupcake molds instead.

Crunchy Lemon Tuna Salad

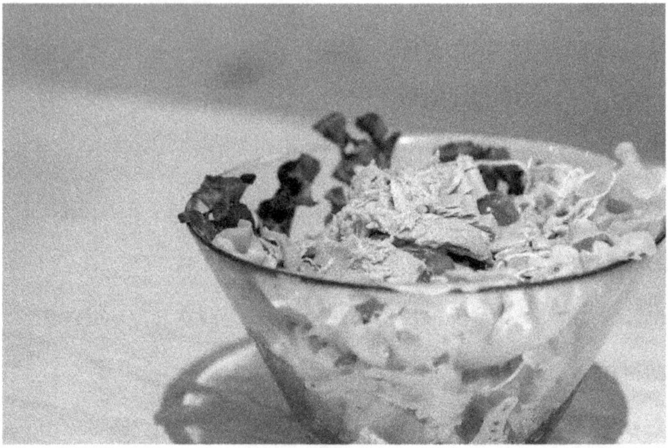

This recipe is actually appropriate for Phase 1 of the Atkins diet, but it's included here to show that, even after you've reached your goal weight, you should still have regular meals that are very low carb and high in protein, vitamins and fiber. Furthermore, tuna is a very inexpensive ingredient that you can make quickly when you don't have time to cook or there's not a lot left in your refrigerator.

Ingredients

5 ounces tuna (canned in water)

1 stalk medium celery

2 tablespoons real mayonnaise

1 cup baby spinach

1 cup arugula

½ onion

½ cucumber

Salt and pepper to taste

1 -2 tablespoons lemon juice

1 teaspoon olive oil

Steps

Step One: Preparing the Tuna

Strain the tuna over the sink to drain the excess water. Place in a medium bowl and add in the lemon juice and mayonnaise. Season the tuna with salt and pepper.

Step Two: Preparing the Vegetables

Chop the celery, onion and cucumber into bite-sized slices. In another medium bowl, mix in the celery, onion, cucumber, spinach and arugula. Toss with the olive oil and more lemon juice if desired.

Step Three: Make the Salad

Portion the salad into a single serving bowl and top with the tuna mixture. Eat immediately or store in the fridge in an airtight container for 3 to 5 days.

Tips

If you need something crunchy, try this salad with a handful of whole wheat pita chips or oven baked kale chips. You can also eat it with whole carrots and celery pieces.

White Bean and Garlic Dip

If you're searching for the perfect savory, creamy dip for your fresh vegetables, look no further than this recipe that combines cannellini beans and garlic to make a delicious mixture that also tastes great as a spread or topping.

Ingredients

1 (15-ounce) can cannellini beans, washed and drained

2 garlic cloves

2 tablespoons lemon juice

1/3 cup olive oil

¼ cup parsley (leaves only)

1 teaspoon rosemary

Salt and pepper to taste

Steps

Step One: Cooking the Aromatics

Heat 1 tablespoon olive oil in a skillet over medium heat. Add in the rosemary and minced garlic cloves. Let them sauté for about one minute before adding in the beans along with salt and pepper. Let the beans heat through for 2 or 3 minutes and then remove from heat.

Step Two: Making the Dip

In a food processor, blend the beans, sautéed garlic, the rest of the olive oil and lemon juice until smooth. Taste and add seasonings as needed.

Step Three: Serving and Storing

Allow to cool and keep in an airtight container for up to 3 days. When serving, top with the parsley leaves.

Tips

Serve this dip at a party with carrots, celery, bell peppers and pita chips. Not only will your guests be impressed, they'll also be enjoying a low-carb dip that's super easy to make!

Thai-Style Chicken Curry with Carrots and Broccoli

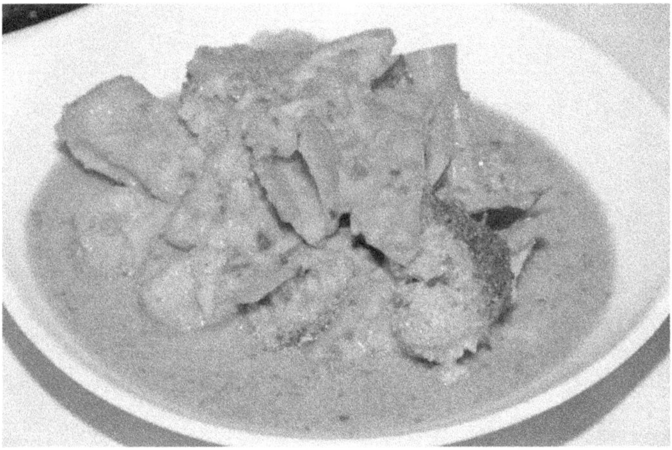

Take chicken and veggies up a notch further with this dynamic Thai-style chicken made with coconut milk and spices. This stir-fry recipe also makes for great leftovers that you can grab while on the go throughout the work week. Try with beef or seafood if you're bored of chicken.

Ingredients

4 chicken breasts, cut into strips

3 tablespoons butter, unsalted

1 teaspoon cumin

½ teaspoon dried coriander leaf

½ teaspoon ground ginger

¼ teaspoon crushed red pepper flakes

2 garlic cloves, minced

½ cup chicken broth

1/3 cup heavy cream or coconut milk

1 bag frozen carrots and broccoli

1/2 lime

Steps

Step One: Cook the Chicken

Heat the butter in a skillet on medium-high heat. Cook the strips of chicken in batches for about 5 minutes until cooked through and browned. In the same skillet, add in the cumin, coriander, crushed red pepper flakes, ginger and garlic cloves. Cook for about 1 minute or until the garlic is fragrant, stirring frequently.

Step Two: Making the Curry

Add in the chicken stock and let the mixture come to a boil. Once it starts boiling, reduce to a simmer at medium-low heat for another 5 minutes or so (cook your vegetables in the meantime). Finally, add in the heavy cream and continue to simmer the curry for about 3 minutes.

Step Three: Cooking the Vegetables

While the curry is simmering, cook the vegetables in a separate skillet according to the instructions.

Once cooked, add into the curry and give the curry a splash of juice from the lime. Serve warm or allow to cool and store in the fridge for 3 to 4 days.

Tips

You can also use jalapeno, snap pea pods, green bell peppers and tomato with this recipe, or whatever frozen veggie mix you have on hand. Of course, this recipe works with fresh vegetables as well (just add in with the chicken stock and simmer until the vegetables are crisp yet tender.

Maple Mustard Baked Salmon with Sweet Potato

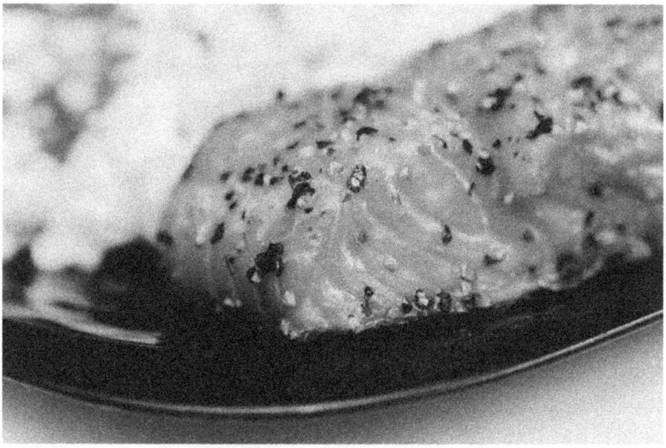

This meal is for that one night a week when you're craving something a little sweeter but want to avoid a fattening meal full of carbs. Salmon is a tasty, fatty fish that contains healthy omega-3 fatty acids. You can flavor it in just about any way you want and it cooks very fast whether it's baked, grilled or sautéed.

Ingredients

For the salmon:

4 salmon fillets

2 tablespoons lemon juice

2 tablespoons Dijon mustard

¼ cup natural or sugar free maple syrup

2 garlic cloves, minced

1 teaspoon lemon zest

Salt and pepper to taste (use crushed black pepper)

For the sweet potatoes:

2 large sweet potatoes

1 tablespoon olive oil

2 tablespoons chopped fresh rosemary

Salt and pepper to taste

Steps

Step One: Making the Glaze

In a medium saucepan mix together the lemon juice, Dijon mustard, maple syrup, garlic cloves, salt and pepper. Let the mixture simmer on medium heat until reduced, 1-2 minutes. Set aside.

Step Two: Preparing the Sweet Potato

Clean the sweet potato and slice into bite-sized cubes. In a medium bowl, toss with olive oil and rosemary.

Step Three: Baking

Preheat your oven to 425 degrees Fahrenheit. On a large baking sheet, arrange the sweet potatoes cubes in an even distribution and bake for 15 minutes. Then, add the salmon to the baking sheet, skin side down. Glaze the salmon with the maple mustard mixture. Bake the salmon and sweet potatoes for about 12 to 18 minutes. You want the salmon to be flaky and the sweet potatoes to be tender.

Tips

Try this recipe with vegetables such as Brussel sprouts and asparagus. You can also use the maple mustard marinade on chicken breast and thighs.

Fruity Turkey Burgers

There's something about eating turkey with fruit that's unique yet enticing for those who enjoy this delicious sweet-and-savory combo. Turkey burgers are a great alternative to beef burgers when you're looking for something a little leaner. Try this turkey and fruit burger recipe – no buns required!

Ingredients

1 pound ground turkey

1 tablespoon olive oil

½ cup red onion, diced

1 teaspoon onion powder

1 garlic clove, minced

½ cup crumbled feta cheese or cubed Brie cheese

½ cup blueberries or cranberries

2 sprigs fresh rosemary

Salt and pepper to taste

Steps

Step One: Forming the Patties

In a large bowl, mix together the ground turkey with the olive oil, diced red onion, minced garlic clove, onion powder, salt and pepper. Fold in the cheese and blueberries or cranberries. Using your hands, carefully form patties and gently push in larger chunks of cheese and berries as needed.

Step Two: Cooking the Burgers

Heat a grill or skillet to medium-high heat. Cook the patties on the grill or skillet for about 5 or 6 minutes per side, or until the meat is cooked through and the juices run clear. Use a meat thermometer to ensure that the internal temperature is 165 degrees Fahrenheit.

Step Three: Serving

Serve the burger patties warm with avocado, lettuce, spinach, arugula and fresh tomato.

Tips

If you feel like you need to have something wrapping the patties, try using lettuce cups, portabella mushrooms, tomatoes, egg plants or red bell peppers. Experiment with different flavors and find something that you enjoy eating while keeping carbs in check. Also try this recipe with ground lamb for something unique.

Dessert

Bittersweet Chocolate Frosted Brownies

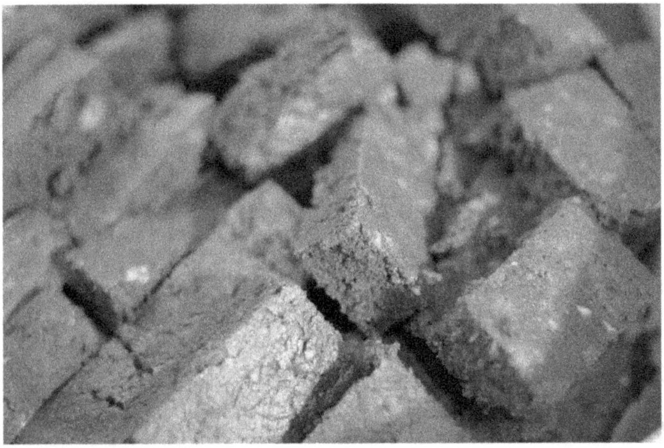

Most of us get chocolate cravings, especially when we happen to be trying to lose weight. Don't worry! With the right ingredients, including unsweetened baking chocolate and full-fat, unsweetened dairy, you can be well on your way to a chocolatey, filling dessert with minimal amount of carbs.

Ingredients

For the brownies:

4 ounces of unsweetened baking chocolate

½ cup heavy cream

5 large eggs

½ cup unsalted butter

1 tablespoon sugar free vanilla extract

1 cup sugar substitute

1 ¼ cups wheat bran or oat bran

2 teaspoons baking powder

½ cup your choice of nuts (optional)

For the frosting:

½ cup dark chocolate chips

2 tablespoons whole milk

2 tablespoons full fat vanilla Greek yogurt (no sugar added)

Steps

Step One: Making the Batter

Microwave the chocolate together with the butter in a microwave-safe bowl for about 2 minutes (don't leave it going any longer than that without checking). Once the chocolate is fully melted, mix in the heavy cream. In another bowl, beat together the eggs with the sugar substitute using an electric mixer. As you're mixing, add in the vanilla extract. Finally, mix in the wheat or oat bran, nuts and baking powder.

Step Two: Baking the Brownies

Preheat your oven to 325 degrees Fahrenheit. Get out an 8 by 8 inch baking pan and spray it with a butter-based cooking spray. Evenly spread the batter into the pan. Bake the brownies until you can insert a toothpick that comes out clean – about 30 to 40 minutes. Remove from the oven and allow to cool.

Step Three: Adding the Frosting

Mix together all the frosting ingredients until well combined. Spread onto the cooled brownies and cut the brownies into bite-sized squares. This recipe makes about 25 brownies.

Tips

You can exclude the vanilla extract if you can't find a sugar free or organic version. Oat bran is a great substitute for flour and contains lots of soluble fiber; however, it's still a carb. Eat this dessert in moderation.

Conclusion

Weight loss is never easy, but following a structured yet flexible program such as the Adkins diet is a great way to get a little help so you can shed pounds and reach your dream goal.

10 Tips for Turning the Atkins Diet into a Lifetime of Healthy Eating and Living

1. Never Starve Yourself

Starving yourself is a sure way to hinder your overall progress to weight loss. Eat when you're hungry (just remember to eat foods that are rich in protein and avoid unhealthy snacks or anything with unhealthy carbs). It is okay to eat lunch early, but never skip breakfast and don't avoid dinnertime either.

2. Always Listen to Your Body

Even if you don't want to use a scale at first, it's important to be able to identify your body's responses to changes in your eating habits and schedule. This is especially important in Phase 2 and 3 because you're trying to determine your ideal carb balance. Keep a journal and write down your weight, how you feel and any changes you notice that could be associated with your diet.

3. Go at Your Own Pace

Everyone loses weight differently. Some people will start seeing results within the first week, while others may take a month or more to experience progress. Factor in how much weight you need to lose and your activity level so you can get a better idea of how you should progress through the phases.

4. Stay Consistent

It doesn't matter how fast you're going, as long as you're going. Plan out your meals for the week by writing them down and always make a list before going shopping, not after. Make it as easy for yourself as possible by pre-portioning your meals and having everything you need at hand.

5. Don't Be Afraid to Ask for Help

When it comes to weight loss, don't be afraid to go it alone. Ask your friends and family to try the diet with you, or at least ask for their support by encouraging them to help you avoid temptations. It's also perfectly fine if you'd like to seek professional help from a nutritionist or a life coach.

Do what you need to do to be the best you that you can be.

6. Start an Exercise Regime that Works for You

The purpose of the Atkins diet is to send your body into fat-burning mode. Even if you hate exercise, try moving your body more by doing aerobic exercises or going for walks. Bring a friend and make a habit of it. The most important thing is that you increase your level of mobility – just keep moving and commit to daily exercise however you can.

7. Get Enough Sleep and Organize Your Schedule

It may be time to make a verbal affirmation that you need to start having a more regular routine. This will help your body adjust to the diet changes, which will therefore allow you to keep better track of your progress. Get as much regular sleep as you can if you need an energy boost.

8. Be Willing to Make Sacrifices

If you're used to eating foods with added sugar and empty calories, the Atkins diet might be a challenge. The great thing about challenges is that they're opportunities to grow and become stronger. You can reduce these types of foods from your diet in a variety of ways; you can go cold turkey, you can slowly reduce them or start using healthier alternatives. Do what works for you and strive for balance and moderation.

9. Make New Goals

Have you finally reached your goal weight? Congratulations! But don't stop there! Keep making new goals. Of course, that doesn't mean "lose more weight". Make a goal for maintaining your weight. Make a goal for meditating or exercising for 10 minutes a day. Make a goal to step up at work and increase your productivity. Whatever it is that you want, make it a goal and go for it.

10. Stay Inspired.

No matter what, don't let go of your dreams. You can adjust or modify your goals, but don't lose sight of what you truly want. Write in a journal, make a blog or create a dream board to help you stay inspired. Surround yourself with positive people and positive thoughts.

I hope that this book has helped give you the tools you need to start taking control of your diet, lose weight and make positive changes to your life, both physically and emotionally. Although this is the end of the book, your journey is only just beginning. Never give up on your goals - your efforts will be met with success!

CPSIA information can be obtained
at www.ICGtesting.com
Printed in the USA
BVHW031157130819
555687BV00002B/129/P

9 781951 339104